W9-BHI-973

Alternative Health Care for Women

A Woman's Guide to Self-Help
Treatments and Natural
Therapies

by

Patsy Westcott and
Leyardia Black, N.D.

HEALING ARTS PRESS
Rochester, Vermont

Healing Arts Press
One Park Street
Rochester, Vermont 05767

Copyright © 1987 by Patsy Westcott and
Leyardia Black, N.D.

All rights reserved. No part of this book may be reproduced or utilized in any form or by any means, electronic or mechanical, including photocopying, recording, or by any information storage and retrieval system, without permission in writing from the publisher.

Printed and bound in the United States.

10 9 8 7 6 5 4 3 2

Healing Arts Press is a division of
Inner Traditions International

Distributed to the book trade in the United States by
Harper & Row Publishers, Inc.

Distributed to the book trade in Canada by Book
Center, Inc., Montreal, Quebec

Distributed to the health food trade in Canada by
Alive Books, Toronto and Vancouver

Alternative
Health Care
for Women

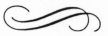

This book is both a
self-help guide and a survey
of therapies particularly
suitable for women.
It includes advice
and information about
preventive health care,
women's illnesses,
fertility and reproduction,
and choosing the best
treatment for you.

Contents

✿ INTRODUCTION—*Women and the Health Services* xi

✿ PART ONE—*Staying Healthy*

A Sense of Well-being	1
Making Changes	2
Back to Basics:	5
You are what you eat	5
Exercise	17
Looking after your body	24
Smoking	30
Stress	32

✿ PART TWO—*Women's Illnesses*

Menstrual Periods and their Problems:	43
What's normal?	43
Lack of periods	43
Heavy periods	45
Menstrual pain	46
Fibroids	49
Endometriosis:	50
Orthodox treatment & diagnosis	49
Alternative treatment & self help	51
Premenstrual Syndrome:	53
The hormonal clue	53
The food connection	54
Who gets PMS?	56
Treatment	56
Headaches and migraine	62

Dealing with anger   63
Vaginal Infections: 65
  Yeast (Monilia)   66
  Trich (Trichomonas vaginalis)   69
  Bacterial vaginal infections (non-specific vaginitis)   69
  Chlamydia   70
  Gonorrhea and syphilis   70
  Alternative medicine and self help   71
  Herpes   72
  Genital warts   76
Other Vaginal Problems: 76
  Cervical Erosion   76
  Bartholin gland cysts and abscesses   77
AIDS (Acquired Immune Deficiency Syndrome)   78
Pelvic Inflammatory Disease   80
Cystitis   82
Benign Breast Disease   84
Cancer: 86
  Breast cancer   86
  Genital cancers   92
  The alternative approach to cancer   95
Mental Health: 103
  The size of the problem   103
  Are you at risk of depression?   105
  What sparks depression?   105
  When to seek help   106
  Orthodox treatment   106
  Alternative approaches to mental health   109

ǯ PART THREE—*Fertility and Reproduction*
Contraception: 111
  Orthodox contraceptive methods   111
  Alternative methods of family planning   115
Infertility: 120
  What are the main causes of infertility?   121
  What treatment is available?   122
  Orthodox treatment   123
Alternative approaches   124

Pre-Conceptional Care   127
Having a Healthy Pregnancy: 128
  What should I eat?   128
  Minor ailments of pregnancy   129·
  Acupuncture for pregnancy and childbirth   134
  Yoga and pregnancy   134
  Osteopathy for pregnancy   135
Birth—Pain Relief: 138
  Alternative and self-help approaches to pain relief in labor 139
  Orthodox methods of pain relief   142
After the Birth—Getting Back to Normal: 143
  Stitches   143
  Breastfeeding   143
  Postnatal depression   144
Menopause: 146
  What signs and symptoms are associated with menopause?   147
  Orthodox treatment   147
  Alternative therapies and self help   148
  Hysterectomy   150

♫ PART FOUR—*The Therapies*
Introduction: 153
  Alternative good, orthodox bad?   153
Finding a Therapist   155
How can Alternative Therapies Help?   156
Nutritional Therapies: 157
  Naturopathy   157
  Megavitamin therapy/Optimum nutrition   159
  Clinical ecology   160
Herbalism   161
  What disorders can herbalism treat?   162
Aromatherapy   164
Bach Flower Remedies   165
Homeopathy   165
  What happens when you visit a homeopath?   166
  How long will it be before I get better?   166
  What disorders can homeopaths treat?   166
  How does homeopathy work?   167

Homeopathy and women	167
Biochemic Tissue Salts	168
Hands-on Therapies:	
Osteopathy	169
Chiropractic	169
Touch for health—applied kinesiology	170
Acupuncture	171
Diagnosis and treatment	173
Shiatsu and Acupressure	175
Reflexology (Zone Therapy/Foot Massage)	176
Massage	178
Alexander Technique	179
Movement Therapies:	181
Yoga	181
T'ai Chi Ch'uan	182
Dance/movement therapy	182
Mind Therapies:	183
Psychotherapy	183
Hypnotherapy	183
Co-counseling—re-evaluation counseling	184
Autogenic training	185
Biofeedback	185
Spiritual healing	186
Meditation	188
Table Showing Illnesses and Therapies	191

Acknowledgements

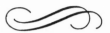

My thanks go first of all to the many alternative and orthodox practitioners who gave freely of their time and expertise during the researching of this book. Next, and no less important, I thank all those friends who shared their personal experiences and views, enduring endless kitchen table discussions that helped enormously in clarifying my ideas.

My thanks, too, to the staff at the Women's Health Information Centre for allowing me the use of their collection; and to Pilgrim Hospital Medical Library, especially Shirley Brewster, for making available many books and articles, and putting up with a chronic late returner.

I'd like to thank Fay Franklin of Thorsons for her patience and support as an editor. And last, but by no means least, I am grateful to my two daughters Lucy and Kate for keeping me going with cups of tea, for putting up with yet another ready meal, and for continuing to love a mother whose mind must have sometimes seemed to be more on homeopathy than the school concert. This book is for them.

Patsy Westcott

While it is not possible to list all of those people who have made contributions to this book, I would like to express my special thanks to Jan Westwater, Licensed Massage Therapist; Cindy Micliu, Licensed Massage Therapist and Acupuncturist; Toni Weschler, Fertility Awarenesss Counselor; Beverly Rackoff, Dance Therapist; Irwin Schiller, Doctor of Osteopathy; Robert Hermer, Counselor; and my patients, from whom I am constantly learning.

I would also like to thank my husband, Charles Black, N.D., for his help, encouragement, and understanding. And finally, thank you to my two-year-old son Aaron for taking three-hour naps.

Leyardia Black, N.D.

Women and the Health Services

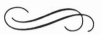

Women are no strangers to the doctor's office. The average woman visits her doctor twice as often, takes more medication, and has more surgery than does the average man.

It's not that we suffer more life-threatening illnesses than do men. Female babies statistically have a better chance of surviving their first year than do males and, in areas where good perinatal care and family planning are available, women, on the average, outlive men by five to eight years.

Some of our visits to the doctor are due to our biology. Our reproductive systems seem to require more upkeep than do men's. Menstruation, pregnancy, childbirth, and menopause may all at one time or another give rise to problems requiring medical attention.

Stress and stress-related illnesses account for an enormous number of women's office calls. The circumstances of many women's lives produce a lot of chronic disability. For instance, although the majority of women now work outside the home, surveys show that most still do the lion's share of the housework, food buying, and meal preparation. Working mothers with children are especially likely to feel that there is far too much to do and too little time to do it in. No matter how hard we work, we feel guilty that we're not doing well enough by our children, home, or job, let alone giving any time to our own well-being. Our guilt compounds the physical and mental stress of trying to do justice to each of these areas in our lives and increases our susceptibility to anxiety, depression, infections, and many chronic diseases—increasing, of course, our visits to the doctor.

Yet, for all the time we spend at the doctor's, we often seem to be dissatisfied with the care we receive. Busy schedules leave many doctors little time to investigate, beyond laboratory tests and physical examinations, the underlying reason for a bout of anxiety or a chronic infection. All too often there is no mention of the possible role that diet, life-style, or emotional issues might play in the patient's present complaint.

Many of us have difficulty in effectively communicating with our physicians. We fail to bring up certain problems or concerns because of embarrassment or the fear that they may seem inconsequential or ridiculous. Women, especially, tend to not be assertive in dealing with their doctors and so may get less satisfaction from their visits than they might.

Also, modern medicine is still largely geared toward dealing with the severely ill patient whose condition is well advanced. It often has no adequate or reasonable treatment for something less than a full-blown disease. A woman with a slightly abnormal Pap test, for instance, is generally told to do nothing more than come back in three to six months to see if the condition has worsened. She is usually not told about any changes she could make in her life or any therapies she might try to improve the condition. She is, however, told that if it does progress some sort of surgery will be necessary to remove the abnormal cells. This situation causes much frustration for many women. They feel that they have lost control and can only wait helplessly to see if things get bad enough to require surgery. This all or nothing approach, here and with many other conditions, leads some women to try alternative therapies.

Another reason women may seek alternative health care is that some of their health concerns may not even be acknowledged by mainstream medicine. Stress- and nutrition-related complaints are often overlooked or misdiagnosed. A woman who sustains a poor diet, alcohol and cigarette usage, and a generally stressful schedule may be dangerously deficient in certain nutrients. Her complaints of fatigue, depression, irritability, and lack of appetite may be seen by a busy practitioner simply as a stress reaction. She goes on her way with a Valium prescription, her severe B-complex deficiency unrecognized and untreated.

This isn't to say that medical heroics aren't sometimes needed or that all medical practitioners overlook life-style and nutrition. There appear to be more and more doctors who do try to take these factors into account and who practice some preventive medicine. Some may also take time to gain some knowledge of alternative therapies and, even if they don't use them in their own practices, might on occasion suggest them as treatment possibilities for certain patients.

Unfortunately, these physicians are still in the minority in most areas of the country, and most patients, women and men, are left to their own devices when it comes to investigating and choosing alternative health care.

So what is alternative health care? What can it do for you? Alternative health care can't work miracles, and you should be extremely suspicious of any practitioner who claims it can. However, it can be an effective first-line treatment for a number of common complaints. It can also be a useful adjunct if you are undergoing conventional treatment.

Alternative health care can help you stay healthy, can treat some illnesses, and can relieve many conditions for which there is no cure. Basic to the alternative health care approach are these ideas:

II The body is finely balanced, and illness is caused when it is out of balance.

II If you become ill, the body has the capacity to heal itself, given the right support and encouragement.

II Disease is often a result of the way we live our lives.

In the following pages we will detail the health problems common to women, examine some of the factors that can provoke a state of illness, and introduce gentle, natural approaches to regaining the health and well-being that accompany a fulfilling life.

Another useful book on women's health to which you might want to refer is *The New Our Bodies, Ourselves: A Health Book by and for Women*, The Boston Women's Health Book Collective (Simon & Schuster, 1985).

PART ONE

Staying Healthy

A Sense of Well-Being

Not only are women the main consumers of health services, they're also the main providers of health care. Whether as nurses, social workers, ancillary workers of all kinds, or as wives, mothers, and daughters, we spend a good deal of time caring for others. But all too often we neglect our own health. We work long hours both outside and inside the home, we rush around trying to fit everything in...and then we smoke, drink, or go on eating binges to cope with all the pressures.

Many alternative therapies are based on the idea that health is damaged by ignoring, repressing, or denying our basic needs. Sometimes it's only when we experience an unexpected miscarriage, a relationship that goes wrong, an illness, or even the development of cancer that we stop short and take a look at our own lives.

That's not to say that it's always your fault if you get sick, nor that you should be in tip-top health the whole time. There's nothing "bad" about being ill. Women blame themselves about enough things without beating themselves over the head for getting sick. In fact, a spell of illness or a bout of depression is the one thing that forces us to take a much-needed break. Being ill can give you breathing space, a time to take stock of who you are and where you are going.

But that said, most of us would prefer to be well. And, though alternative health care can't solve the problems of insufficient money, pollution, where you live, the work you do, and many of the other causes of ill health, it can help you to take care of yourself so that you are better able to withstand disease. You don't have to wait for your health to break down to make changes in your life. You can start now to tune in to your own physical, social, and spiritual needs. Alternative health care means paying attention to what you eat, getting enough exercise, feeding your mind, and feeling a sense of fulfillment in life.

In a world where women in particular suffer from a lack of choice and power, looking after your own health and knowing when to seek help can give you a valuable sense of control. It can also give you extra energy and confidence to get involved in practical things that might change life for the better, if you wish, for both yourself and others.

The idea most of us have about health is that it is an absence of illness. But how many of us who aren't exactly ill can say that we feel really healthy either? A whole Pandora's box of aches and pains, headache, depression, palpitations, indigestion, rheumatism, chronic tiredness, high blood pressure, and sore throats is opened when women are asked about their general condition. The fact is that many of us feel slightly under par much of the time. And while illness is part of the normal flux of life, many of us experience an ebbing of vitality and a lack of "zest." A sense of well-being can be yours whatever your age or disabilities. It comes from knowing who you are and where you are going.

Making Changes

Change calls for action. So how do you start? The first step is to take a hard look at your life. The key to health from this perspective lies in giving due weight to all the different aspects of your life. That means not only taking care of your body by attending to what you eat, getting enough exercise, and so on, but also looking at your social relationships, your mental life, and your spiritual needs. This last is quite difficult for most of us to understand. Traditionally, such needs have been the province of religion. With the decline in church-going and organized religion, the spiritual dimensions of life have tended to be ignored or dismissed as irrelevant. But whether you subscribe to an accepted faith or not, the truth is that we all need to make sense of our lives and to feel a sense of direction and purpose.

Ready ...

Start off by imagining how you would like your life to be if you had completely free choice. This is your first taste of a technique called visualization, or guided meditation. Don't censor yourself at this point. If you've always had a fantasy of going off and living on a Greek island with a couple of goats for company, go ahead and indulge in it. You'll be able to work out what's realistic and what isn't later. But you can't decide how to achieve what you really want until you know what it is.

... Get set ...

Once you've thought about how you would like your life to be, you can start to inject some realism into your program. It may help at this point to write it all down. Set yourself goals. Say what you would like to be doing in five years' time, one year, six months, and three months. This will help you plan and, more important, it will help put time under your control. Not having enough time to do what we want to do is one of the major causes of stress—and of ill health.

Be specific and try to get a balance between the various different areas of your life. For instance, don't just say "I want to get more exercise," say "I'm going to go swimming every Tuesday evening between 7 and 8 p.m."

... Go!

Once you've got your plan of action you can start to put it into practice. You're more likely to succeed if you bear the following tips in mind:

✵ Be realistic. If you don't have proper training or don't have child care, you may have to wait to get that perfect job. However, you could begin working toward it by checking child care options in your area and by taking courses in your field of interest. In the meantime, is there anything else that would satisfy that need—for instance, getting involved in a community group?

✵ Be practical. Unless you're very self-disciplined you're not going to trek across town on a winter evening to that yoga class. Is there anything nearer home you could do?

✵ Know yourself. Take into account your own strengths and weaknesses. Are you the sort who will stick religiously to a jogging routine, or would you be better off trying to do some other sort of exercise two or three times a week? For further ideas on this see the chapter on exercise.

✵ Take it a step at a time. Even positive changes like going on a vacation are stressful. Don't let getting healthy become another stick with which to beat yourself.

✵ Be prepared for setbacks. You're bound not to meet your goals from time to time, so be kind to yourself. If you constantly fail to reach a target it's not because you're no good. Perhaps you're being too ambitious. Could you do something different, or break down what you've set yourself to do into smaller, simpler steps?

✵ Get others in your life on your side. If you've decided to set aside twenty minutes a day for meditating, arrange for

your partner, a friend, or a neighbor to look after the children, organize a game for them, and make sure they understand that you are not to be interrupted.

✍ Beware of becoming a fanatic. Start slowly.

✍ Live in the present. Begin by making small changes that you can easily make right now. And don't wait to start living until you've got a better job, stopped smoking, started exercising, or whatever.

✍ Learn to listen to yourself. Be aware of your own feelings. Your dreams, intuitions, tastes, and preferences—what you like and dislike—are all important messages about you. With practice you can use them to guide you into making the right choices for you.

Body

What is right for you in the way of diet and exercise? See the sections on these for some ideas. Are there any health problems that need attention? What alternative therapies might be able to help you? See Parts Two and Four for hints on these. Beware of becoming what holistic doctor Laurence LeShan calls a "holistic athlete," jumping from one therapy to another in the hope it will solve all your problems. Remember, true change can only come from within you.

Mind

Many of us take it for granted that our mental powers will automatically deteriorate as we get old. Yet research shows that using the brain cells actually stops them from degenerating. Even those of us who are in good physical shape may neglect our mental well-being. Don't. For others the approach to physical health can be made via the mind. For ideas on this see the section on mind-body therapies.

Relationships

Research shows that women are at more risk of depression if they don't have a close, confiding relationship. Improving the quality of your relationships may mean discussing with a partner what you really want from your partnership, and reassessing other relationships that have become stale and dead. It can mean recognizing the ways in which you yourself contribute to rigid patterns. It may even mean breaking out of a relationship that has become dull and stultifying, or deciding to make changes in it.

Deciding to seek psychotherapy, joining a co-counseling group, or exploring other alternative therapies can help you to be clear about some of these points.

Spirit

Specific techniques such as yoga, T'ai Chi, or creative activities such as dance, drama, music, art, and writing can help create a sense of greater awareness and meaning in life.

Although I've divided all these areas up for the sake of convenience, they don't exist in isolation. Your aim is to achieve a balance in all areas of your life. The next sections will help you do this.

Barriers to change

It isn't always easy to change. Habits and patterns of behavior build up gradually over long periods of time. Other people's expectations of how women should live their lives often lie at the root of our problems. The fashionable ideal of the perfect figure forces us to starve ourselves and contort our shape. Images of the perfect wife and mother isolate many women in the home. Fear that we're the only ones who shout at our children, stick them in front of the television, or feed them junk food cuts us off further from others in the same situation.

Making changes involves a degree of risk, too. And many of us have a lot invested in staying the way we are. It only takes a child to say "I don't like it now that you go to evening class" to make most of us crumple. Keeping a sense of balance helps, and so does not trying to do too much at once. Meeting and talking with other women does also. Find out if there's a women's health group or other women's group near you. We'll be looking some more at some of these barriers to change and how you can overcome them in the mind-body section of the book.

Back to Basics

You are what you eat

The food we eat is one of the cornerstones of alternative health care. The role of diet in chronic and degenerative disease, allergies, behavior problems, and a whole host of other nasties has been exhaustively chronicled. What's perhaps less well publicized is why so many of us find it hard to follow all the good advice.

Women are the great providers. We're the ones who, on the whole, buy, prepare, and cook most of the family's food. But despite all this it's one of the areas in which many of us feel particularly out of control. And feeling out of con-

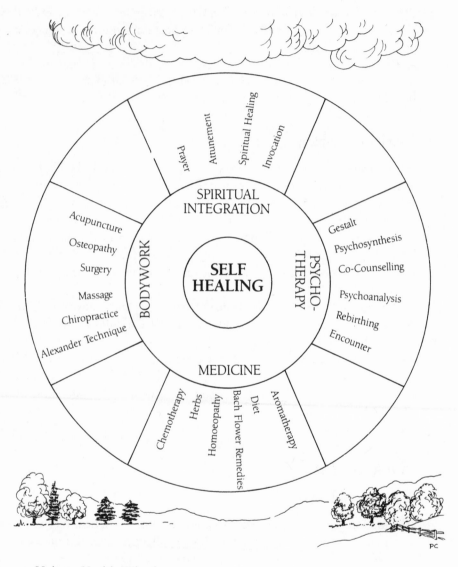

Holistic Health Wheel

Alternative health care means seeing yourself as a whole.
You need to think about all these areas of your life.

trol is one of the major sources of stress, which in turn is believed by many alternative practitioners to be the root of most illness.

On the one hand, we're bombarded with advice on what we should eat. On the other, millions of dollars are poured into persuading us to buy products, many of which are patently unhealthy. At the same time we have to juggle the competing demands of different family members and make it all fit the budget.

A report from York University showed that for many families a "proper meal" is still meat and two vegetables, with desserts a reward for cleaning your plate. And, despite women's liberation, many of us are still caught up in the idea that the way to a man's heart is through his stomach. Add to this the fact that the kids won't eat anything unless it's fried or smothered in ketchup, and that you are on a diet, and it's small wonder that family meal times are the traditional time for bickering!

For many women their role as provider and consumer of food is tied up with feelings of who they are. The women in the York study saw it as their job to prepare the meals and do the dishes. What's more, if you're at home all day, preparing and serving dinner may be one of your few creative outlets. If the family turn up their noses at what you've spent hours lovingly slaving over a hot stove making, it's hardly surprising if you feel a failure. Food then is often a measure of our "success" as wives and mothers. And if you're dieting, resisting tempting goodies becomes a measure of your "success" as a woman. So you can see that there's far more to food than having a good diet.

So what's wrong with the food we eat nowadays? And what can you do about it? Although there seems to be more choice than ever before, it is often between one variety of junk food and another. You've only to examine the shelves of the local supermarket to see just how much of what we eat is processed in some way. Buying whole foods and additive-free products usually means paying more. And even those that are labeled "additive-free" may have hidden preservatives—in the flour, say, of an "additive-free" pizza. The good news is that some stores are bowing to consumer pressure and stocking organically grown vegetables and fertile eggs, albeit at somewhat inflated prices. One way around this is to buy in bulk, or to see whether there are any food co-ops in your area.

To supplement or not to supplement?

The fact that we all eat too much fat, refined sugar, and starches, and too little fiber and fresh fruit and vegetables, can hardly have escaped anyone's notice in the last few years.

In the last fifty years or so, a complex food industry has grown up, making available a whole range of foods that take up less shelf space, keep longer, and take less time to cook. The problem is that processing destroys many essential nutrients. Many alternative practitioners and nutritionally oriented therapists argue that because of this and modern methods of factory farming, even those of us who are apparently well fed could be short of essential vitamins and minerals. Even fresh foods, they say, are low in nutritional value. They may be contaminated with lead from the atmosphere or aluminum from cooking utensils, all of which can lead to deficiencies and excesses of vitamins and minerals that cause all manner of diseases (for more about this see specific illnesses in Part Two). The answer, according to these experts, is vitamin and mineral supplements.

The whole question of supplementation marks the great divide between orthodox doctors and many alternative practitioners. Conventional dieticians and nutritionists, and some naturopaths, claim that as long as you are getting a balanced diet there's no need for supplements. Supplements, too, are big business, as you can see if you wander down the aisle of your local health food store.

But the supplementation story is far from clear-cut. A lack of vitamins and minerals may well cause deficiency diseases, but an excess can actually be harmful. The efficacy of megadoses of vitamin C, for example, once hailed as the great cure-all for everything from the common cold to cancer, has been challenged. What's more, too much vitamin C may lead to kidney stones in susceptible people, and can cause withdrawal effects if used for more than one or two weeks. (If you are taking large doses, wean yourself gradually.) And megadoses of vitamin C in early pregnancy have been found to put women at greater risk of miscarriage.

Methods of testing for vitamin and mineral deficiency or excess are fraught with all sorts of difficulties, not the least of which is that no one seems to be able to decide what the recommended daily allowances should be. And in many cases we don't know whether a disease or condition causes deficiency or whether it's the other way around.

Finally, nutrients don't work in isolation. Vitamin C, for instance, is needed for iron absorption. Zinc and vitamin A work together. Adding extra vitamins or minerals willy-nilly can throw the body out of balance. Any supplement you take needs to be carefully tailored to you as an individual.

It's all very confusing, isn't it? So should you supplement or not? The box shows times when you might be short of certain nutrients. If you think you need a supplement consult a practitioner with a special interest in nutrition.

Do I need a supplement?

If you think you may need a supplement the following guide can help you decide. Women who may need extra vitamins or minerals are:

☞ Those who eat an unbalanced diet—for instance, if you're a strict vegan, hate raw vegetables, or are excluding certain foods from your diet because of allergy.

☞ Those who are dieting, especially if overall intake is below 1,200 calories a day. If you're dieting you may well be low in vitamins A, C, B_6, calcium, iron, and magnesium.

☞ Those who have heavy periods. You may need extra calcium because of the risk of osteoporosis (see menopause section). This should be taken with magnesium to make calcium intake more effective. You may also be in need of extra iron.

☞ Those who smoke or drink heavily. In this case you will probably need extra vitamin C, vitamins B_6 and B_{12}, thiamine, riboflavin, folic acid, magnesium, and zinc.

☞ Those who are pregnant and breastfeeding. For further details see the chapter on pregnancy.

☞ Those who are over sixty, especially if you are eating a restricted diet because of lack of money, disability, or ill health.

☞ Those who have to take regular medication for a chronic ailment; for instance, cortisone can rob the body of calcium.

If you regularly take over-the-counter medicines (aspirin, for instance, increases the body's need for folic acid, vitamin C, and iron).

The Pill can cause a shortage of B_6.

☞ If you've recently been ill or are convalescent. Certain illnesses and infections can rob the body of nutrients.

Rules for taking supplements

☞ Don't take isolated vitamins or minerals without the advice of a qualified practitioner.

☞ Always take the supplement with your meals.

☞ If you buy a multi-vitamin/multi-mineral supplement choose one with a wide and balanced variety of nutrients.

☞ Don't expect vitamins and minerals to make up for poor eating habits.

☞ If in doubt consult a qualified practitioner.

Healthy diet guidelines

So what should you eat? And how do you ensure that you are getting a healthy diet? The following guidelines will help you find your way through the diet maze. We've also included a list of minerals and vitamins so you can see what they are and what they do. If you try to choose as varied a diet as you can you shouldn't go far wrong.

⌇ Increase your intake of whole-grain cereals, brown rice, whole-grain bread, whole-grain or buckwheat pasta.

⌇ Eat plenty of fresh fruits and vegetables.

⌇ Eat more raw food—some experts claim that 60 percent of our diet should be raw.

⌇ Avoid storing food for too long. Fruit and vegetables lose nutrients very quickly and other foods can develop harmful organisms the longer they are stored.

⌇ Cut down on animal fats found in red meat, hard cheeses, and so on.

⌇ Choose white meats such as chicken and game animals, e.g., rabbit.

⌇ Buy oils high in polyunsaturates such as sunflower, walnut, and safflower. Cook in more saturated oils such as olive oil, rather than fat.

⌇ Cut out fried foods. Broil, steam, or stew instead.

⌇ Avoid sugary foods—cookies, cakes, sweets.

⌇ Eat more fish. Fish is low in fat, and fish oils seem to protect against heart disease. Recent evidence suggests that a diet high in fish oils may help prevent premature births.

⌇ Eat more vegetable proteins such as beans, chick peas, nuts, and seeds. Incidentally, the protein value of legumes is increased by combining them with a grain product, e.g., lentils and brown rice.

⌇ Don't re-use cooking oils.

⌇ Cut processed foods of all kinds to the very minimum.

⌇ Drink less coffee, tea, cocoa, and soft drinks. The caffeine in these can make you edgy as well as prevent the body from absorbing certain nutrients (vitamin B_1—thiamine). It's also, according to some practitioners, a factor in hypoglycemia (low blood sugar), which is responsible for making us feel low.

⌇ Drink more herb teas, fruit juices, bottled water.

Changing to a healthier diet will be easier if you go slowly. Try out new foods when you are feeling relaxed. If you lead a busy life—and who doesn't—invest in a pressure cooker. This takes a lot of the time out of cooking legumes. If you can afford it, a freezer and a microwave oven are also invaluable. Finally, remember, *how* you eat is almost as important as *what* you eat. Eat your meals in a relaxed frame of mind.

Additives

As women, the additives problem affects us particularly. Additives have been blamed for birth defects, stillbirths, and lowered fertility. Women working in the food-processing industry in Finland were shown in one study to have a higher risk of miscarriage. And we still don't know how today's plethora of additives might affect future generations.

What's more, the foods liked by kids—chips, jelly, ice cream, candy, and soda drinks—are some of those highest in additives. Children may be especially at risk from their harmful effects. Their immature immune systems mean they are less able to cope with poisons, which, in their smaller bodies, may have a greater effect. Eczema, asthma, diabetes, hyperactivity, diarrhea, stomach pains, tantrums, rhinitis, mouth ulcers, vaginal discharge, and miscellaneous aches and pains are just some of the complaints blamed on additives by some researchers.

Apart from these specific problems, additives can affect your body's ability to absorb nutrients from food. Some additives can destroy vitamin B_1, essential for a healthy nervous system. Others bind to nutrients such as iron and calcium so that our bodies are unable to use them. Small wonder so many complaints can be traced back to the food we eat. And all this can be seen as further evidence of the lack of control we have over our lives.

So what can you do if you are worried? On an individual level, eat as much fresh and unprocessed food as you can, and read labels. There are now several books on the market (see the following). You can badger your supermarket and food manufacturers to provide additive-free foods; bring the matter to the attention of any groups you belong to, and write to your congressman. At present there are many research projects going on into the effects of additives on our health. In the meantime—watch that label!

For further information:

A Consumer's Dictionary of Food Additives, Ruth Winter (Crown Publishers).

Nontoxic and Natural, Debra Lynn Dadd (Jeremy P. Tarcher, Inc.)

Irradiation—a new peril?

The furor over additives has caused manufacturers to look to new ways of preserving food. In Holland and elsewhere, high intensities of X rays are used to prevent fresh food from deteriorating. At present this has limited use, but there are signs that the use of irradiation in food preservation may increase.

Irradiation reduces the nutritional value of foods. A subcommittee of The Advisory Committee on Irradiated and Novel Foods in Great Britain discovered losses of vitamin B_1 (thiamine), folic acid, and vitamins C, K, and E. What's more, irradiation may affect the composition and taste of food so that further additives are necessary.

Even more worrisome is the suggestion that food may be at greater rather than less risk of being contaminated because of irradiation. This is because the process can mask signs that food is going bad. It also produces chemical substances, called radiolytic products, that aren't naturally present in foods. We don't really know what the effects of these are.

What foods will be affected? The main ones will be cereals, spices, fruits, vegetables, chicken, shellfish, and other meat.

For further information:

> The National Coalition to Stop Food Irradiation
> P.O. Box 59-0488
> San Francisco, CA 94159
> Phone: (415) 566-2734

> Health and Energy Institute
> 236 Massachusets Ave. N.E. Suite 506
> Washington, D.C. 20002
> Phone: (202) 543-1070

Food Irradiation: Who Wants It?, Tony Webb, Tim Lang, and Kathleen Tucker (Thorsons).

Becoming a vegetarian

Vegetarians usually enjoy excellent health. Vegetarian women are at less risk of breast cancer. And cancer of all kinds seems to be less common in people who don't eat meat. There's also evidence that a vegetarian diet can help improve menstrual problems, especially if it contains a larger number of raw foods.

A recent study by an Australian team of naturopaths looked into the nutritional status of the "new vegetarians," people who had chosen to become vegetarian for health reasons. They looked at life-style, nutrition, and level of illness, and carried out blood and biochemical tests. The "new vegetarians" were well supplied with vitamins C, B_2, and beta carotene (which may explain why there are fewer cases of cancer among vegetarians). But women especially were low in iron and vitamins B_1 and B_{12} (the lack of which can cause irritability and depression). Those most at risk tended to eat more junk foods—even though they were vegetarians. The moral seems to be to eat a good, balanced diet, taking special care to get enough vitamins and minerals. And if you do suffer any troublesome symptoms, see a nutritional specialist to see if you could benefit from a supplement.

For further information, contact:

> Baltimore Vegetarians
> P.O. Box 1463
> Baltimore, MD 21203
> Phone: (301) 752-VEGV

> North American Vegetarian Society
> P.O. Box 303
> Burton, WA 98013

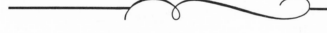

YOUR GUIDE TO VITAMINS AND MINERALS

A (fat soluble)

Sources: Liver, cheese, eggs, carrots, green leafy vegetables, tomatoes, dried apricots, oily fish
Why you need it: For healthy bones and teeth, better eyesight, helps resist infection, helps you resist cancer, protects mucous membranes.

B_1 Thiamine (water soluble)

Sources: Brown rice, whole-grain cereals and breads, pork, liver, peas, seeds, nuts, molasses, brewer's yeast
Why you need it: Helps digestion, healthy blood, muscle tone, eyes, heart, hair, brain and nervous system, and helps inhibit pain.

B₂ Riboflavin (water soluble)

Sources: Spinach, leafy green vegetables, eggs, whole grains, brown rice, meat, cheese, liver, kidney, fish, brewer's yeast
Why you need it: Healthy eyes; healthy skin; helps your body process protein, carbohydrates, and fats; cellular respiration.

B₆ (water soluble)

Sources: Liver, beef, oily fish, whole-grain products, wheat germ, walnuts, peanuts, prunes, avocados, raisins, bananas, leafy green vegetables
Why you need it: Helps fight infection, helps your body use magnesium and linoleic acid, helps in sodium/potassium balance of body. Especially useful for a number of women's menstrual problems and those connected with menopause. Healthy blood, nerves, muscles, and skin.

B₁₂ (water soluble)

Sources: Kidney, liver, heart, eggs, herrings, mackerel, cottage cheese
Why you need it: For cell growth, helps iron function in the body, processing of fats, carbohydrates, and proteins in diet. Healthy blood and nervous systems.

Folic acid (water soluble)

Sources: Leafy green vegetables, liver, kidney, brewer's yeast
Why you need it: For healthy blood (prevents anemia), glands, and liver; helps circulation and cell growth; and stimulates appetite.

Niacin (water soluble)

Sources: Wheat and whole-wheat products, peanuts, fish, liver
Why you need it: Helps circulation, helps reduce cholesterol. Healthy hair, brain, heart, and other internal organs. Aids production of sex hormones.

Pantothenic acid (water soluble)

Sources: Liver, kidney, eggs, cheese, mushrooms, elderberries
Why you need it: Helps body deal with stress, helps it make use of vitamins. Healthy adrenal glands, digestive system, immune system, nerves, and skin.

C (water soluble)

Sources: Green vegetables, potatoes, citrus fruits, blackcurrants, berries
Why you need it: Helps digestion, aids healing, prevents bleeding, helps resist coughs and colds and other infections. Healthy adrenal glands, blood, blood

vessels, skin, bones, teeth, and gums. Especially necessary if you smoke, drink, or are under stress. Some experts claim it can help treat cancer.

D (fat soluble)

Sources: Eggs, liver, oily fish, fortified milk, sunlight
Why you need it: Helps your body absorb calcium and phosphorus, important if you are to avoid osteoporosis (brittle bones) in middle age. Helps heart to pump, maintains nervous system, aids blood clotting. Healthy bones, heart, nerves, skin, teeth, thyroid.

E (fat soluble)

Sources: Eggs, cereals, peanuts, fruits, nuts, vegetable oils, soybeans
Why you need it: May delay ageing, reduces cholesterol levels in blood, improves blood flow, possible aid to fertility. Healthy blood vessels, heart, lungs, nerves, skin, and pituitary function.

K (fat soluble)

Sources: Lean meat, liver, green vegetables, cereals, molasses, yogurt
Why you need it: Healthy blood, blood clotting, healthy liver function.

Calcium

Sources: Sardines, soy, milk, cheese, yogurt, watercress, molasses, nuts
Why you need it: Healthy blood, bones, teeth, heart. Especially important for avoidance of osteoporosis (brittle bones) in middle age. Helps calm nerves, regulates heart and acid/alkaline balance of body.

Chromium

Sources: Brewer's yeast, whole grains, liver, cheese, molasses
Why you need it: Healthy blood and circulation, helps balance blood-sugar level, and regulates energy levels.

Copper

Sources: Lobster, nuts, raisins, wheat germ, olives, molasses, oysters
Why you need it: Helps hemoglobin formation, helps regulate emotions. Healthy blood, skin, nerves, hair, bones.

Iodine

Sources: Fish, seafood, kelp
Why you need it: Regulates thyroid activity, helps produce energy. Healthy hair, nails, skin, teeth.

Iron

Sources: Meat, liver, eggs, sardines, legumes, oats, whole-grain bread, figs, prunes, dried apricots, molasses
Why you need it: Formation of red blood cells, helps resistance to stress. Healthy blood, nails, bones, skin.

Magnesium

Sources: Meat, poultry, fish, nuts, bran, milk, green vegetables, whole-grain flour, brown rice, brewer's yeast
Why you need it: Acid/alkaline balance of body, energy metabolism, aids proper utilization of calcium and Vitamin C, may help prevent PMS (premenstrual syndrome). Healthy blood vessels, heart, muscles, teeth, nerves.

Phosphorus

Sources: Meat, milk, eggs, grains, yellow cheeses
Why you need it: Bone and tooth formation, cell growth and repair, helps body use vitamins and absorb sugar and calcium. Healthy bones, brain, nerves, muscles, teeth, kidneys.

Selenium

Sources: Fish, whole grains, brown rice, nuts, brewer's yeast, broccoli
Why you need it: Helps pancreas to work properly, may help fight cancer. Healthy tissues.

Potassium

Sources: Meat, vegetables, dates, figs, peaches, molasses, peanuts, raisins, bananas
Why you need it: Helps calm you down, controls heartbeat, muscle contraction. Healthy blood, heart, muscles, nerves, kidneys, skin.

Sodium

Sources: Salt, milk, cheese
Why you need it: Regulates fluid levels in cells, prevents cramps. Healthy blood, muscles, nerves, lymphatic system.

Zinc

Sources: Beef, liver, seafood, oysters, nuts, cheese, whole-grain bread, ginger, mushrooms, sunflower seeds

Why you need it: Helps healing of wounds, helps digestion of starchy food, may help avoid anorexia (not proved), counters depression, aids metabolism of B_1, phosphorus, and protein. Healthy blood and heart, healthy sex organs.

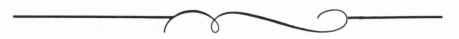

For further information:

Nutrition Almanac, John D. Kirschman (McGraw-Hill).

Exercise

Exercise makes you look and feel better. It puts a spring in your step and a glow in your skin. It helps keep your weight under control, reduces your chance of a heart attack, and helps you sleep better, eat better, and feel less depressed. It tones up your muscles and gives you more stamina. Exercise helps you cope with stress. So why don't more of us do it?

One reason perhaps is that women are brought up to think of themselves as passive and weak. Athletic ability is associated with being unfeminine. And even the frenetic jogging and working out of the current fitness craze seems to have at least as much to do with the attainment of an unrealistic female shape as with the health benefits. What's more, if you're unused to it, exercise hurts! Your muscles feel sore, your joints ache, and at least to begin with you feel older and more liable to fall to pieces than ever.

However, it's well worth persevering because the right kind of exercise really can help you withstand stresses and strains more easily. The secret is to choose a form of exercise that suits you. If you enjoy it you're more likely to stick with it. There are innumerable forms of exercise to choose from. And one advantage of the fitness boom is that so many different sorts of exercise are available wherever you live. Which should you choose? Ask yourself these questions:

- How much time do I have to spare?
- How much money can I afford?
- Would I like to exercise on my own or with others?
- What's available in my area?
- What are my particular physical strengths and weaknesses?
- What sports or physical activities did I enjoy at school?
- What sports or physical activities do I enjoy watching?

If you're not the athletic type, some of the movement awareness techniques such as yoga, T'ai Chi, Alexander technique, or dance may suit you better than taking up a sport. If you dislike the jock image of sports there are plenty of other ways to exercise, either alone or in company.

If the social side is important to you, join a fitness class or gym if you can afford it. If you feel embarrassed at the thought of working out with men, find one that holds women-only sessions. Incidentally, when you first start to exercise, doing it with a friend can help keep up flagging motivation when it starts to hurt, or when staying home seems more appealing than going to your workout.

If you are busy, choose something that will fit easily into your working day, or you'll be tempted to give up. How about bicycling to work? Swimming during your lunch hour? Going for a workout immediately after you finish work?

If you've got small children you could choose an exercise that will involve them, too. Local pools may hold "duckling" sessions for toddlers. Alternatively, choose a daytime class with day care, if there is one in your area, or get a babysitter and get completely away for one evening a week.

If you prefer exercising alone, then running, swimming, walking, and bicycling are good all-round choices.

Starting to exercise is the hardest step. Once you've started to feel the benefits you won't want to give up.

The three main aims of exercise are to build up strength, mobility, and stamina. Observe the following rules and you'll soon begin to reap the benefits of being fitter:

✍ Always spend some time warming up and cooling down.

✍ Choose an exercise you think you'll enjoy. You can use the visualization technique described on page 2 to help you decide what possibilities there might be.

✍ Try to exercise at least three times a week.

✍ Work up gradually—don't overstrain yourself. "Going for the burn" can be positively harmful.

✍ Find out as much as you can about particular exercises, what parts of your body are used, whether it's aerobic (i.e., designed to increase oxygen intake and therefore energy), and so on. Then try to choose a series of exercises to provide a balance.

✍ If you develop physical signs such as ulcers, sore throats, sleeplessness, and fatigue, you could be overdoing it. Stay in touch with your body and know when to stop.

♫ Exercise will often improve menstrual problems, but if you are suffering badly from PMS or pain it may be better to delay exercising until you feel better. A relaxation session instead may be what you need to put you in a better frame of mind. Be guided by your body. See the section on menstrual problems (page 43) for more suggestions.

WHICH EXERCISE

Walking

Cost: Low. You don't need any special equipment beyond a pair of good strong shoes and something waterproof in case it rains.
Suitability: Suits all ages and states of health. Can be fitted easily into your everyday life if you're very busy.
Advantages: Exercises your heart, burns up energy, yet is gentle and nonstressful. Helps clear your mind. Some claim to reach an almost meditative state while walking.

Swimming

Cost: Low.
Suitability: Suits all ages and levels of physical fitness. Can be useful if you suffer from a heart condition (always consult your doctor first), are overweight, or have arthritis. Available wherever you live.
Advantages: Good for posture. Exercises most of your major muscles, including the heart. Has been called the best all-round exercise. You can pace yourself. Helps relaxation. Water is soothing, especially the sea. Good if you're pregnant, as the water takes your weight.

Bicycling

Cost: A good bike can be fairly expensive, but it's a once-only expenditure. If you plan to take up bicycling seriously, you may want to join a club and buy special clothing (which will increase cost).
Suitability: Good for any age. If you have children you can all bicycle together.
Advantages: Once you've learned the basics you can bicycle almost anywhere, though town bicycling is not always pleasant or safe. Good for your heart and lower limbs. Doesn't do a lot for your upper body. Good way of meeting people if you join a club. Risks of back injury, heat, and cold. Wear correct clothing and a helmet, and pay attention to how you ride.

Dance

Cost: Varies according to where you go and what type of dance you choose. Leotards, tights, and so on can all mount up.

Suitability: Anyone of any age or state of fitness can do it. Women especially often feel a real affinity for dance. Find out about different types; for instance, belly dancing is a wonderful, sensuous form of dance especially suited to women—even a round stomach is an advantage!

Advantages: Allows you to express emotions in movement. Increases flexibility, develops leg muscles. Good way to meet others. Some type of dance likely to be available wherever you live.

Running/jogging

Cost: Cheap, though running shoes can be expensive and you should select the best you can afford.

Suitability: Any age; you can do it anywhere, any time, which makes it especially useful if you're busy and don't have much time.

Advantages: Exercises your heart, lungs, and legs. Good for meeting people if that's what you want, or you can do it alone. Runners "high" releases endorphins into system, giving sense of well-being. Running is not for everyone and may cause knee and foot problems. Check with your physician before beginning.

To decrease possible exercise related injury see: *Stretching*, Bob Anderson (Shelter Publications).

Exercise in pregnancy

Exercise in pregnancy can increase your strength and suppleness so you are better able to cope with the extra demands on your body. It can also help you cope better with labor—though it can't guarantee you an easy birth. It helps you relax and combat sleeping problems, and gives you a feeling of well-being. Dance is an especially suitable form of exercise if you are pregnant. Many communities offer special dancing classes for mothers-to-be. Be sure to follow these guidelines for safe exercise in pregnancy.

✓ Check with your medical advisor before embarking on an exercise routine.

✓ If you're not used to exercising, go gently, and stop if you feel any pain.

✍ Don't wear yourself out.

✍ Choose non-weight-bearing exercises such as swimming, bicycling, or stretching which doesn't have bouncing actions. Ease off exercise other than stretching in the last four weeks.

✍ Avoid surfing, windsurfing, mountain climbing, skydiving, and other dangerous activities. Sports or exercises involving precise balance and coordination may be more risky as your center of gravity changes and your sense of balance may be affected.

✍ Exercise regularly so long as pregnancy is straightforward, but no sudden bursts.

✍ Exercise for shorter periods and take regular rests in order to maintain blood supply to the baby.

✍ Take your pulse every ten to fifteen minutes. If it rises to 140 a minute slow down until it is 90 or under.

✍ Don't get too hot. If your baby gets overheated it can cause developmental problems, especially during the first three months. Avoid exercising for longer than half an hour at a time if it's hot or muggy.

✍ Cut down on hot baths and saunas.

✍ Rest for ten minutes lying on your left side after exercise to allow your body to recover.

✍ Drink two or three glasses of water after exercising to replace fluids lost through sweating. Drink whenever you feel thirsty during exercise. Increase the amount you eat to replace calories burnt off by exercise.

✍ Increase the amount you eat to replace calories burnt off by exercise.

✍ Stop exercising immediately if you get out of breath, feel dizzy or numb, or experience pins and needles, pain, or bleeding. Consult your doctor.

For further information:

Weight Control in Pregnancy Dr. Jennifer J. Ashcroft and Dr. R. Glynn Owens, (Thorsons).

Don't neglect your pelvic floor

Your pelvic floor is the hammock of muscle that lies between your pubic bone and your lower spine. The muscles form a figure eight around the bladder, uterus, and bowel and hold them in place. You use them when you are making love to squeeze your partner's penis or fingers, during childbirth to allow the baby to emerge smoothly, and to control the flow of urine.

Sometimes the muscles can become slack and flabby. This can be a result of too little exercise, too hard pushing during childbirth, overweight, a job that involves a lot of heavy lifting, and simply age, which reduces the amount of estrogen in your system. If you lose tone in your pelvic floor, you may suffer any or all of the following:

🍋 a lax vagina with less sensation

🍋 prolapse of the uterus (when your uterus drops out of place)

🍋 inability to fully empty your bladder, leading to increased urine infections

🍋 constipation

🍋 stress incontinence, i.e., leaking of urine if you laugh, sneeze, cough, or run

🍋 fatigue after standing for too long, and a heavy dragging feeling as if your "insides are falling out."

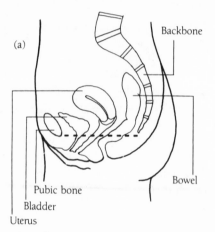 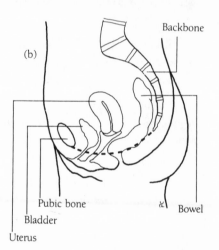

Pelvic floor conditions.
(a) Position of organs in the body with good pelvic floor support. (b) With poor support the organs descend and the pelvic floor sags.

Fortunately, it's possible to improve your pelvic floor muscles at any age. The secret is pelvic-floor exercises (sometimes called Kegel exercises). These are invisible exercises that you can perform any time of day, when you are talking on the phone, waiting in a line, or whatever. They involve tightening and lifting the pelvic floor.

Identify the muscles by trying to stop the flow of urine. If the muscles are weak, you may have some trouble doing this. Don't persist until you have built up some strength, as you may weaken them even further. You can also identify the muscles by trying to grip one or two fingers placed in your vagina, either your own or your partner's, or your partner's penis. If your muscles are strong your partner will wince with pleasure...this is known as positive feedback! Don't worry if contractions get weaker as you continue squeezing—it's perfectly normal.

THE EXERCISES

1. Tighten up the whole pelvic floor and hold it for three seconds, relax. Repeat five times. Do this several times a day, working up gradually until you are doing about ten sets of these exercises a day. If your muscles feel sore, temporarily reduce the number of exercises to allow your muscles to recover.

2. Imagine that your pelvic floor is an elevator; gradually raise it to the first, second, third, fourth, and fifth floors, stopping briefly on each one. Then go down again gradually. Always tighten your pelvic floor at the end of this exercise. After all, you wouldn't walk around with your mouth hanging open, would you, so why do it with your pelvic floor?

3. Draw up and relax your pelvic floor quickly, as though pumping water in and out of your vagina.

Don't overstrain yourself, and work up gradually. And always remember to tighten your muscles at the end of each exercise.

Benefits of looking after your pelvic floor

         a better sex life

         helps your body cope better with the stress and strain of pregnancy and birth

         helps avoid stress incontinence

Incidentally, some evidence suggests that *any* exercise, not just those aimed specifically at this area, can improve pelvic floor tone.

If you do suffer from a weak pelvic floor, osteopathy may be able to help by correcting imbalances in posture that may have affected the muscular hammock. Yoga exercises are also beneficial, and you'll find several suitable ones in *Yoga in Pregnancy* by Vibeke Berg (Watkins).

Finally, your pelvic floor may be weakened if you have a persistent cough, so try to get this cleared up. Avoid constipation by eating a high fiber diet. And if you are experiencing pelvic floor symptoms such as those mentioned earlier, which don't go away despite a concentrated program of pelvic-floor exercises, see your doctor, as you may need surgery or treatment such as a special ring pessary to support the uterus.

♫ Looking after your body

Your breasts

Many of us feel discontented with our breasts. We feel they're too small (usually) or (more rarely) too big. This is hardly surprising given the fact that a pair of "perfect" breasts can be used to sell almost anything. Becoming familiar with our breasts can help us learn to like them and accept them as part of ourselves, whether they are firm or soft, big or small. Examining your breasts can also help you detect any small changes that may be a sign of cancer or benign breast disease at an early stage.

Advantages of examining your breasts:

> ♫ You become familiar with what they
> feel like at different stages of your cycle

> ♫ Nine out of ten breast lumps are discovered
> by women during self-examination

When should you do it? Your breasts will be easier to examine and less lumpy immediately after your period.

How to do it

1. Stand in front of a mirror with your arms by your sides, and look at your breasts. You're looking for any changes in texture such as dimpling or an orange peel appearance. There's a wide variation in women's breasts. If you've had a baby, been on the Pill, or lost a lot of weight you may be able to see little silvery ridges that are stretch marks.

2. Next lie down. Place a cushion or towel under your shoulder and feel firmly but gently. A circular motion is best, moving from breast bone to the nipple, around it and under your arms. If you're unsure of how to do it, ask a doctor or nurse, at the family planning clinic, for example, to show you how. Make sure that you examine each part of your breast.

3. Repeat on the other side.

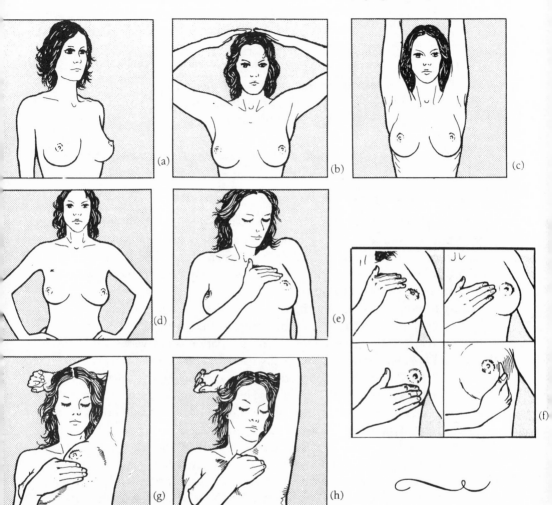

Breast self-examination.

(a) Look at yourself in a mirror. (b) Put your hands on your head and look for any irregularities, especially around the nipples. (c) Stretch your arms above your head and look again. (d) Repeat this procedure, this time with your hands on your hips. (e) Lie on a flat surface with your shoulder slightly raised by a towel. Feel your left breast with your right hand, using the flat part of your fingers. (f) Working in a circle, feel every part of your breast. (g) With your left arm behind your head, repeat the circular movement, especially around the outer part of the breast. (h) Finish by feeling the tail of the breast, toward the armpit. Repeat with the other breast.

What you are looking for

Any changes on the surface of your skin or deeper lumps. Most lumps turn out to be harmless. A fluid-filled mass that feels like a peeled grape will usually be a cyst; a fatty tumor that hurts when you squeeze may be a fibroadenoma. The sort of lump to be most suspicious of is a hard mass that doesn't move and seems to grow into the surrounding tissue or be anchored to the chest wall.

If you find any sort of lump, though, you should see your doctor to put your mind at rest.

To screen or not to screen

Conventional wisdom says we should each examine our breasts every month. However, unless you've been taught how to examine yourself properly there's no guarantee that you will detect a lump earlier than you would through casual handling. In the meantime you may have subjected yourself to a process which has made you extremely anxious.

Massive health education campaigns to get us all to examine ourselves have been singularly unsuccessful. Why? One expert writing in a medical magazine points out that psychologically, breast self-examination is not very satisfying: the "reward" you get for doing it is the discovery that you have a serious, and sometimes fatal, disease. Some authorities point out that by the time a lump is large enough to be felt it will usually have been there for some time. What's more, some large lumps are very slow in growing, while some small ones are of an aggressive type that gets worse very quickly.

So what should you do? The answer seems to be that if you feel secure examining your breasts, go ahead and do it. On the other hand, if the whole process distresses you and you decide not to do it, you aren't necessarily reducing your chances for successful treatment, *if* you have your breasts clinically examined every year and include regular mammographic examination after age forty.

Mammography

Screening with mammography (a breast X ray) can detect a lump before it is big enough to feel.

The newer mammography machines emit an extremely low dose of radiation. When used in conjunction with a specially designed diagnostic ultrasound, mammography can allow a trained radiologist to see lumps as small as 1 mm in diameter. It can also help predict whether the lump is cystic or solid, which can help direct further diagnosis and treatment.

Mammography alone may be all that is needed to accurately image the breast in a woman over fifty who has a high ratio of fat to glandular tissue in her breasts. In younger women with denser breast tissue, the use of diagnostic ultrasound in conjunction with the mammography helps define areas which might not show up well with mammography alone.

In addition to finding lumps, these techniques can tell what basic type of breast tissue a woman has: fatty, dense, dysplastic, etc. Knowing this can help a physician predict a woman's likelihood of developing breast cancer in the future. At this time, the American Cancer Society recommends that all women have a baseline mammogram between ages thirty-five and forty, followed by annual or biennial mammograms from age forty to forty-nine, and annual mammograms from age fifty on. In view of the high predicted incidence of breast cancer in women (one in eleven), and the relative safety and accuracy of new diagnostic techniques, this recommendation seems reasonable.

The rate of breast cancer has increased significantly over the last forty years. While improved early diagnostic techniques can increase survival from minimal breast cancer to 90 percent, the fact that one in eleven women can be expected to develop it in the first place is cause for concern. Obviously we need to be looking for more ways to prevent cancer, and this is where alternative medicine can come in.

Down below

There's one part of our bodies about which most of us are completely ignorant, despite the fact that it plays such an important and fundamental part in our lives—our genitals. We allow our most intimate orifices to be explored by our lovers, or the doctor's rubber-gloved fingers, but the majority of us have no idea what we look like "down below."

Becoming familiar with this part of your body can be an important part of getting to know yourself. Each of us is different, just as the noses on our faces are all different. It can remove the mystery from our genitals and help us feel more at ease with our sexuality. It can help you spot any potential health problems, such as an erosion or infection, at an early stage so that you can begin treatment or seek help. You will be able to detect any changes earlier than a doctor who only examines you occasionally. It can help you to take control of your own fertility by practicing natural family planning methods.

Some women examine themselves together with other women in a women's health group, as part of the process of demystifying gynecological care and getting to know their own bodies. But there's no reason why you shouldn't examine yourself at home.

What you will need

✍ a flashlight or Tensor lamp

✍ a mirror

✍ a plastic speculum—this is the beak-like instrument doctors use to do an internal examination. Your local women's group or women's health group might sell them.

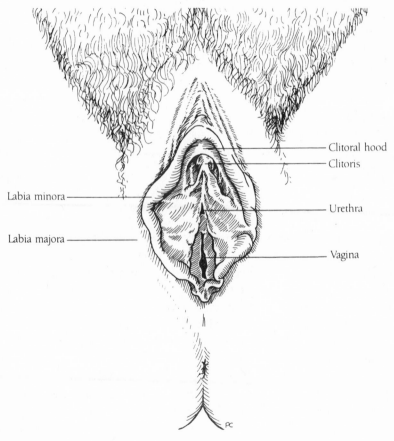

The external female sex organs.

WHAT YOU CAN EXPECT TO SEE

1. Start by examining your outer genitals. You'll see the fatty pad called the *mons veneris*, covered by pubic hair. In some women the pubic hair can extend some way up the abdomen, and down onto their thighs. The hair covers the outer lips of your genitals—the labia majora.

2. Next, using the mirror if necessary, explore between the outer lips. You'll see the inner lips (labia minora). These can be anything from pinkish to purplish-brown in color, and may look thin and ragged or plump. When you are sexually aroused they become swollen, increasing sensation.

At the top, inside your inner lips, you'll find your clitoris. It's a small pink "button" partly covered by a hood of skin, and is exquisitely sensitive. In fact, it's the heart of women's sexual arousal.

Spread the inner lips and you will see below your clitoris the urinary opening, and below that your vaginal opening. This is normally closed, but stretches and fans out like a flower during sexual arousal or childbirth. If you are a virgin and have never used tampons you may find the vagina covered in a thin membrane called the hymen.

3. Now you're ready to look inside your vagina. Insert the speculum gently and lock it open. You'll see your cervix or neck of the womb, like a shiny rosy knob with a dimple in the middle—the *os*. If you've had children this will be slightly wider. You'll notice your vaginal secretions, and will be able to tell if you have an infection (see pages 65-76).

4. If you see a reddened shiny area on your cervix, this is probably an ectropion or erosion. This can be caused by a variety of factors—being on the Pill, recent childbirth, irritation from an IUD (coil), or hormone imbalance. In most cases it can go without treatment, but it would be wise to see the doctor for a check up (see also pages 76, 77).

5. If you examine yourself at different times in your cycle you'll notice your cervix and vaginal walls change in color and texture. Your cervix also gets higher or lower depending on where you are in your cycle.

6. It's best not to examine yourself during pregnancy. Once you've tried self-examination you may want to make it a regular part of your health care routine, or you may feel satisfied to leave it to the medics. But whether you do it once or adopt self-examination as a regular practice, it can be an enormously enlightening and exciting experience.

For further information:

The New Our Bodies, Ourselves: A Health Book by and for Women, The Boston Women's Health Book Collective (Simon & Schuster).

SELF-HELP HEALTH CARE GROUPS

Many women in various parts of the country have set up self-help health groups. The idea is to share information and experiences, to demystify health care, and to provide a different way of looking at health care and caring for our bodies.

Such a health group may be held in someone's home, a women's center, or a health or community center.

The National Womens Health Network, 224 7th St. SE, Washington, DC 20003, has information about groups throughout the country, or you might be interested in forming one of your own. Activities and subjects that might be included are:

- Self-examination
- Menstrual problems
- Birth control
- Childbirth
- Sexuality
- Cancer
- Menopause
- Alternative therapies

Above all, such groups are positive and practical.

Smoking

Lung cancer seems about to replace breast cancer as the number one cancer killer for women. Smoking is strongly linked with cancer of the cervix. If you take the Pill and smoke you have a three times higher risk than normal of getting heart disease. Smoking has been associated with early menopause. And if you smoke while you are expecting a baby, you're more likely to suffer a miscarriage, give birth to a low-birth-weight baby, and experience problems during pregnancy and labor.

Barriers to giving it up

Antismoking propaganda is a classic bit of victim blaming—it's *your* fault if you smoke and it serves you right if you get any of the diseases I've already mentioned. The finger of blame is especially pointed at mothers-to-be who smoke. But all this condemnation ignores one fact—the reason people smoke in the first place. Research shows that women have special difficulties in quitting. Why?

Lighting up a cigarette can be a safety valve. It helps you calm down and reduces tension that you feel you can't get rid of in any other way. One woman quoted in a book on women's health says: "If a guy's fed up he can walk out of the door. You can't because of the kids and so you light up a cigarette."

Another woman in the *The Ladykillers: Why Smoking Is a Feminist Issue*," by Jacobson (Pluto), a study of women smokers, says: "I don't want to scream and yell and hurt people so I smoke."

What's more, those around us can actively sabotage our efforts to stop. If we are nasty or irritable it isn't unknown for a member of the family to go out for a pack of cigarettes "to stop Mom being bad-tempered."

Having a cigarette is also a way of breaking up the day or relieving boredom. Women who are anxious, worried, or depressed, or who are in stressful jobs, smoke for similar reasons.

A big barrier to giving up for many women is the fear of putting on weight. Smoking calms the appetite and can be a nonfattening alternative to a visit to the cookie jar.

In a leaflet published by the Women's Health Information Centre, England, the point is made that many women find it hard to stop smoking because we're not brought up to focus on long-term goals. Much of our lives consists of filling in time in the short term: waiting to get married, to have a family, for the kids to grow up, the phone to ring. This particularly relates to the fear of getting fat if we give up smoking: "The effect that excess weight will have on her life and self-image can seem a greater threat than contracting a disabling disease many years in the future."

Much of cigarette advertising is aimed at women, with smoking portrayed as sophisticated and glamorous.

Giving it up

♬ Eating more fresh fruits and vegetables helps you give up smoking, according to a study from the Department of Psychology at New Columbia University. Apparently, fruit and vegetables make the body more alkaline, thus making it expel nicotine more slowly; by reducing the rate at which nicotine leaves your body, it extends the time before you need your next "fix."

♬ Take up exercise. As we've already

seen, exercise releases endorphins, giving you a sense of well-being that may reduce the nicotine craving.

🥢 Join a self-help group, or give up smoking with a friend or partner.

🥢 Hypnosis and acupuncture can both be beneficial; hypnosis by its relaxation effect, and acupuncture possibly by its endorphin-releasing quality. But, as an acupuncturist warned, "It can't enable someone to give up if they don't really want to."

🥢 Learn to relax. (See page 38.) But relaxation on its own isn't enough. Smoking is not just a chemical addiction, it also has to do with the way you live.

Become aware of the times when you feel the need to smoke and plan ahead so as to avoid or cope with them. The stress reduction techniques outlined in the following section will come in handy here. Simply learning how to view a stressful situation in a different light may help. Psychotherapy which uses "cognitive restructuring" techniques can be useful here.

🥢 Alter your routine. Take up knitting, join a group, read a book, play with worry beads...anything to take your mind off the dread weed.

🥢 Avoid smoky places and atmospheres, as well as situations in which you would normally smoke.

🥢 Stress

It may seem odd to include stress in a chapter on how to stay well. Nonetheless, learning how to deal with stress is one of the most important ways in which we can help ourselves to stay healthy. With increasing research it appears to be the linking point between alternative and orthodox approaches, and may provide the key to how and why so many of the alternative therapies work.

There's hardly an illness in existence that doesn't involve a large dose of stress. Indeed, many alternative practitioners and not a few orthodox ones would claim that stress lies at the root of most ailments. Even so, stress is an inescapable part of life. As stress expert Hans Selye has said, "Complete freedom from stress is death." It's worth bearing this in mind since we so often think of stress as an entirely bad thing. A certain amount of stress gives us the get-up-and-go necessary for living. It can also be a useful pointer. It can provide the impetus for change and can give us the motivation and insight into things that are bothering us so that we can take action. However, severe, prolonged stress is dangerous. It affects every system of our bodies and can lead to serious illness.

Women's lives, women's stress

Sources of stress come from outside and from within. Living in today's world we are exposed to noise, pollution, traffic, and over-crowding. At the same time, we often feel isolated, trapped in our own homes without the intimate relationships that can support us and sustain us in the face of day-to-day difficulties. Of course, most of these outside stress factors affect men too, but women are exposed to the additional effects of these stressors by virtue of living in a man's world.

If you are a mother with small children, you have to face the daily aggravation of living in a world where children are at best tolerated as a nuisance, at worst totally ignored. Try struggling to the store with a baby or toddler in tow, fighting your way through swinging doors too narrow for a stroller, not to mention the hassle of public transportation, for starters.

If you work outside the home, you may have had to face barriers in getting the sort of job you want, lack of training opportunities, and discriminatory attitudes. You may have to work part-time in a badly paid job with unsociable hours because of lack of training or because it's the only job that fits in with family commitments.

If you're trying to juggle home and work there are even more stresses. Women are the ones who overwhelmingly make and maintain child care arrangements. You're probably knocking yourself out to prove you're as good as the next one at work, then rushing home to cater to the family. Despite ideas of equality, old habits die hard, and women still carry the main burden of looking after home and family. Lack of official recognition of the needs of families, limited child care facilities, subtle and not so subtle pressure to conform to certain images of women can all make us feel guilty about working outside the home at all. This is despite the fact that four times as many families would be below the poverty line were it not for wives' wages. The stereotype of the high-powered career woman who puts the demands of the board meeting before the needs of her children serves to perpetuate and obscure the real issues. And it all adds up to further stress.

When you add on the stresses connected with the biological milestones that punctuate our lives—menstruation, pregnancy, menopause—it's hardly surprising that so many of us fall prey to stress-related disorders.

The message put out by doctors, the media, employers, and others around us is that everyone should be stable and rational at all times. If we are not we risk being labeled "ill" or in need of treatment. Perhaps the fact that nine out of ten of us suffer mood changes connected with our menstrual cycles should prompt the questions "What is normal?" and "Who says?"

Nonetheless, the interaction of such social, psychological, and biological factors in the face of expectations of others adds up to a big stress potential.

Large numbers of us feel, and in fact have, little control over our lives. And for most of us stress is long-term. It's these two factors—lack of control and prolonged stress—that experts believe are so debilitating to health.

Under stress

What happens when you are under stress? Quite simply, the body prepares to cope with the threat to its equilibrium by the familiar "fight or flight" mechanism. In physical terms, the hormones adrenalin and nonadrenalin are released into the bloodstream, causing the following:

⌨ Your heart beats faster.

⌨ Your blood pressure rises.

⌨ Your breathing gets faster and lighter.

⌨ Your muscles tighten, ready for action.

⌨ Your mouth becomes dry (saliva dries up).

⌨ Your digestive system closes down so that blood can be diverted to other parts of the body.

⌨ Your pupils get bigger.

⌨ Your liver releases sugar into the system to give you extra energy.

⌨ Your urine output is affected as a result of blood flow to the kidneys being reduced.

⌨ Your immune system shuts down.

It's hardly surprising, where the body is under continual stress, that these powerful effects can take their toll on your health. The physical effects of stress have an additive effect if they go on for any length of time—high blood pressure can lead to heart problems, constant release of acids into the stomach leads to stomach problems such as colitis, irritable bowel, diverticulitis, ulcers, and so on, and when the immune system closes down, your body is less able to deal with infection.

Are you under stress?

Check any symptoms you regularly experience.

☐ Headaches

☐ Dry mouth

☐ Sweaty palms

☐ Dizziness

☐ Rashes

☐ Panic attacks or anxiety

☐ Problems relaxing

☐ Mind constantly on the go

- ☐ Yawning or sighing
- ☐ Swallowing difficulties
- ☐ Palpitations
- ☐ Sexual problems
- ☐ Indigestion
- ☐ Irritable bowel
- ☐ Menstrual problems
- ☐ Bursting into tears
- ☐ Aches and pains in the muscles, e.g., your shoulders, back, stomach
- ☐ Execessive drinking or smoking
- ☐ Loss of appetite
- ☐ Compulsive eating

- ☐ Exhaustion even after a good night's sleep
- ☐ Sleeping difficulties—sleeping either too little or too much
- ☐ Lack of concentration
- ☐ Irritability
- ☐ Anxiety about your health
- ☐ Muscle twitches
- ☐ Low self-esteem
- ☐ Lack of concentration
- ☐ Loss of interest in life
- ☐ Cold hands and feet (through poor circulation)

Adding up the stress factors

Psychologists Thomas Holmes and Richard Rahe discovered a link between the number of stressful events in your life and emotional and physical health. To assess this, they developed a stress scale. How does your life add up?

Useful though it is, there are one or two points worth bearing in mind about this scale. The scale reflects dominant social values such as the importance of marriage as a source of stability. In fact, marriage itself can be a source of stress and ill health for women. And though there's no denying the pressures on women when a relationship has broken down, often linked with the material disadvantages they suffer, research has shown that single women are far healthier than single men, and that married women are unhealthier than married men.

Women may be especially at risk of stress from relationship breakdown because for many of us our identity is tied up with other people. Try writing down ten sentences beginning with the words "I am" and see how many of them relate to you as an appendage of the others in your life.

Second, it's hard to disentangle the effects of stress, such as increased smoking, drinking, poor eating habits, and all the habits that we may adopt in an effort to cope with stress, from the stress itself. And as you'll see in the rest of the book, these in themselves can affect our ability to withstand disease.

Working out your stress score			
Death of your partner	100	Change in responsibilities at	29
Divorce	73	work	
Marital separation	65	Children leaving home	29
Jail term	63	Trouble with in-laws	29
Death of close family member	63	Outstanding personal	28
Personal injury or illness	53	achievement	
Marriage	50	Spouse begins or stops work	26
Fired from your job	47	Begin or end school	26
Marital reconciliation	45	Change in living conditions	25
Retirement	45	Change of personal habits	24
Change in health of a	44	Trouble with your boss	23
member of your family		Change in working hours or	20
Pregnancy	40	conditions	
Sex problems	39	House move	20
New family member	39	Change in schools	20
Business readjustment	39	Change in leisure	19
Change in financial state	38	Change in church-going habits	19
Death of close friend	37	Change in social life	18
Change to different line of	36	Medium mortgage or loan	17
work		Change in sleeping habits	16
Change in number of arguments	35	Change in number of family	15
with your partner		get-togethers	
Large mortgage	31	Holiday	13
Foreclosure of mortgage or loan	30	Christmas	12

Score over 300 and you stand an 80 percent chance of coming down with a physical illness in the next year.

Finally, if you're worried or upset you may be more inclined to visit the doctor with symptoms that you might otherwise ignore. Women especially find it hard to ask for help, and visiting the doctor can be a way of getting the nurturing and attention you feel unable to ask for in any other way.

That said, there's no doubt that stressful events do play a role in illness.

For instance, one study found that the husbands of women who had recently died of breast cancer had severely lowered immune response for some time afterward. Looking at the stress scale it's not hard to see how a cascade of stress can occur. Take a pregnancy for example. Chances are this will lead to changes in your sex life, your financial state, your working habits, job, sleep, eating habits, and quite a few others. The point is, it all adds up to stress.

How can you help yourself?

A large part of this book comes down to helping yourself deal with the effects of stress. So what can you do? Experts in stress reduction say a two-fold approach is most helpful:

1. Anticipate stress.
2. Develop a battery of coping strategies to help you cope with unavoidable stress.

Let's take pregnancy as an example again. Although motherhood is held up as the highest achievement we can reach, it's also downgraded in the status stakes. Anticipating stress can mean writing down all your fears and worries about becoming a mother, however trivial, and using your list as a basis for discussion and action. If you are worried about birth, for instance, you can make it your business to find out about local hospital policies and methods of pain relief, get information on how to help yourself, and sign up for a course of prenatal classes. This last will put you in contact with others undergoing the same experience—a valuable counter to stress. A similar action plan can be useful for any stressful situation.

Another useful technique is "noticing." Instead of being waylaid by all the thoughts and feelings that fill your mind, make a point of paying attention to what is going on around you. Concentrate on your physical surroundings, the process of doing whatever you are engaged in at that moment, so as to be truly aware.

Coping with stress

- Expect change and accept it as normal.
- Don't hang on to the past.
- Accept yourself as you are.
- Don't do something just because you feel it is expected of you.
- Learn how to say no.
- If you have a problem, talk about it.
- Find something absorbing to do—work or a leisure activity, anything that engages your whole attention.

⫿ Give yourself a break. Spend time doing nothing, reading, walking, having a bath, anything you enjoy.

⫿ Hang on to your sense of humor—it really is the best medicine.

⫿ Get some exercise—physical activity releases stored-up tension

⫿ Learn to relax.

⫿ *Don't* drink more, smoke more, or take drugs.

Basically, what this all comes down to is looking after yourself—something women often find hard to do.

⫿ Alternative therapies

Virtually all the alternative therapies can help you deal with stress. The key is to find the one that suits you. Going to see an alternative practitioner can be something you are able to do for yourself, and can improve self-esteem. It can also give you the energy to deal with stressful situations.

Psychotherapy, co-counseling, and other mind-body therapies can help identify the roots of problems. They can allow you to express emotions such as anger, fear, and sorrow safely, without the consequences they might have in real life.

Meditation, yoga, and T'ai Chi can help you relax and slow down your body and mind, giving you a break from problems and reducing the harmful bodily effects listed earlier. In fact, in a study carried out at the University of Arkansas College of Medicine, meditation was shown to have a direct effect on the immune response mechanism.

Learning to relax is something positive you can do for yourself. Anyone can do it, and you don't need special equipment.

1. Choose a time when you know you won't be interrupted, and take the phone off the hook.

2. Loosen any tight clothing, then sit or lie down.

3. Tighten each muscle in turn, working from the toes to the top of the head.

4. Now loosen each muscle, letting each one become as floppy as you can, and feel your body become heavy.

5. Stay like this for ten to fifteen minutes, breathing slowly and calmly. If any disturbing thoughts occur, as they will, simply let them flow in and out of your mind. It can help to focus your mind on a soothing scene, or concentrate on your breathing or heartbeat.

With practice you will be able to relax easily any time you want. Practice relaxation once or twice a day, and use the routine whenever you need to calm yourself during the day, for instance, if you have a difficult meeting, exam, or whatever.

Learn to assert yourself

Many of us have difficulty in asserting ourselves and find ourselves doing things we don't really want to, or living up to other people's expectations of us instead of our own. This often arises out of the "good girl" syndrome, in which we spend our lives pleasing other people in order to be liked. Learning to say no calmly and to ask for what you want without getting upset or feeling guilty is the essence of assertiveness training. It can help give a sense of greater control over life, which leads to a reduction in stress.

The secret of saying no without feeling guilty is to acknowledge certain basic human rights. These include the right to be treated as an intelligent, capable, and equal human being, to change your mind, to express your own opinions even when they conflict with those of other people, to ask other people to meet your needs, and to decide whether or not to respond to theirs. Can you think of any others? Recognizing your own rights involves acknowledging those of others too, of course. And it doesn't mean getting your own way all the time. Flexibility and being able to see another's viewpoint are also important.

Being assertive doesn't mean being aggressive or unreasonable. It means being able to ask for what you want calmly and honestly without becoming angry or upset and with respect for others.

Assertive skills can be useful in all sorts of everyday situations, and also in more specific ones like childbirth, dealing with the medical profession, or dealing with your partner. The techniques are simple to learn, though you'll probably learn better in a group, where you can practice, rather than from a book.

Breathing

Hyperventilation or overbreathing is the cause of many problems. Shallow, fast breathing is a result of stress and can also increase anxious feelings. Learning to breathe slowly and calmly can help reduce tension and make you feel more energetic.

1. Sit or lie in a relaxed position.

2. Place a hand on your upper chest and one on your stomach.

3. Breathe in slowly until your bottom hand rises. If you're doing it properly the upper hand should barely move.

4. Hold your breath for a count of five, then slowly breathe out. Pause, then repeat again.

5. Repeat ten times.

You can use this exercise to calm yourself if you are feeling tense, to get to sleep, or before practicing meditation or relaxation.

Sleep

Anxiety can be the biggest reason for not being able to drop off at night, or perhaps you are having pain from a chronic illness.

☞ Start to wind down a couple of hours before bedtime. Read a book, practice your yoga, or meditate.

☞ Avoid stimulating discussions or arguments.

☞ Have a warm bath. Add aromatic oils such as lavender, chamomile, marjoram, sage, rose, ylang ylang.

☞ Get a partner or friend to give you a massage.

☞ Drink an herb tea such as valerian or chamomile to calm your nerves. You can buy special mixtures from the health food store that are combinations of relaxing herbs.

☞ Use an herb pillow.

☞ Listen to a relaxation tape or play a favorite piece of music.

☞ Avoid eating too late at night, and avoid coffee, tea, alcohol, or other stimulants.

☞ If you can't get to sleep, spend the time drifting, practicing visualization, or meditating to refresh and revive you. Experts think that we only need about five or six hours of sleep anyway, and an occasional broken night never hurt anyone in the long run. You'll be better able to withstand it if you have spent the sleepless hours relaxing.

☞ Above all, don't panic, and try to avoid tranquilizers and sleeping pills.

Avoiding work stress

🖎 Pay attention to lighting. The best type of lighting is that which is comfortable for the job.

🖎 Don't sit for too long—it can hamper circulation. If you can, get up and walk around every hour or so; otherwise tap your feet.

🖎 Pay attention to your seating. If the seating is too high, use a footrest or a pile of books to raise it to a comfortable height.

🖎 Don't stand for too long.

🖎 If you work with video display units make sure you have regular breaks, and don't work on one for too long, especially if you are pregnant.

🖎 Make sure there is adequate fresh air. Plants, flowers, and bowls of water will moisten the air. An air ionizer will reduce stuffiness.

🖎 Develop assertive skills to deal with your superiors.

Of course there's not always a lot you can do on an individual level about poor working conditions. Working together with others will help.

If you feel your physical health may be especially sensitive to something in the workplace, contact the Human Ecology Action League, Inc., 7330 North Rogers Ave., Chicago, IL 60626. They should be able to put you in touch with groups in your area who can help.

For further information:

Successful Stress Control: The Natural Way, David Hoffmann (Thorsons).

PART TWO

Women's Illnesses

Menstrual Periods and Their Problems

Forty out of every thousand women visiting the doctor each year go with menstrual problems, and many more simply suffer in silence. Not many of us believe nowadays that we'll turn the milk sour, make bees die, rust iron or brass, or stop the bread from rising when we have our periods! But too many of us are ignorant about just what is normal during menstruation, which makes it hard to know when and where to seek help.

☿ What's normal?

One way to become familiar with your own individual pattern is to keep a menstrual diary. The variation in "normal" is enormous, and the twenty-eight-day cycle is a bit of a myth. Most of us, in fact, experience irregularities in cycle length, amount of bleeding, and so on throughout our lives. Many menstrual problems that have no apparent cause result from stress interfering with hormone balance. This chapter looks at what menstrual problems you might experience and what you can do about them. However, do bear in mind that most alternative therapists don't look at symptoms in isolation, and so will probably not use the conventional classifications outlined here.

☿ Lack of periods (amenorrhea)

The most common reasons for not having periods, of course, are pregnancy and breast-feeding. Doctors conventionally define two types of amenorrhea: primary, when your periods have never started, and secondary, when they have been apparently normal and then stop. In practice, the boundaries between these two are not that clear-cut. Given the enormous range in cycles in those of us who are perfectly healthy, unless you go three or more months between periods and/or you are trying to conceive, there may be no need to seek help.

When to seek help

If you haven't started your periods by the time you are eighteen you may need special tests to see what is causing the delay. Quite often, the reason is stress or other emotional upsets. Very occasionally amenorrhea is a result of congenital abnormalities for which, sadly, little can be done by orthodox or alternative medicine. In this extremely unlikely event there will usually be several other signs that something is wrong.

Hormonal disturbances affecting the thyroid, extreme weight loss (for instance, if you are anorexic), drugs such as those used to treat high blood pressure or cancer, coming off the Pill, and a few rare diseases such as pituitary tumors are the most common medical reasons for lack of periods.

Women athletes who train heavily may often have irregular periods or no periods at all. In this case, amenorrhea appears to be associated with loss of bone mass which in turn can lead to osteoporosis. Women athletes who experience amenorrhea should seek advice on how to moderate their diet and exercise to regain their periods.

Conventional treatment

Conventional treatment consists of tests to find out why you aren't having periods, plus hormone treatment or drugs to stimulate the hormone producing centers in the brain, such as Clomid, a drug used to treat infertility. Very occasionally, if the cause is thought to be psychological, you may be offered tranquilizers or antidepressants.

Alternative treatment and self help

Herbal treatment is extremely effective for amenorrhea, though a qualified herbalist advises against treating yourself. Garden sage (*Salvia officinalis*) is useful in regulating your periods. A number of herbs can be used to rebalance your hormones, where this seems to be the underlying reason for the problem. Chaste tree, also known as monk's popper (*Vitex agnus castus*), is particularly useful.

Homeopathy is a useful first line of treatment where there are no obvious physical causes. Acupuncture is also useful. If you are using alternative therapy, make sure you are also using contraception, since if you suddenly ovulate you could become pregnant.

For stress relief try biofeedback and meditation, plus the stress coping measures outlined in the previous section.

Since amenorrhea is so tied up with infertility, you'll find further details on alternative approaches in the section dealing with fertility and reproduction.

ℐ Heavy periods (menorrhagia)

Again it's difficult to say what is normal, since the amount of blood loss varies from woman to woman and throughout life. You will know what is normal for you. If you pass large clots or soak the sheets at night, or blood gushes through clothing in the daytime, then seek help.

The commonest reasons for excessive bleeding are hormonal imbalance, IUDs, fibroids or polyps, endometriosis, obesity, certain rare blood diseases, stress, and very occasionally, cancer. You'll find some of these dealt with elsewhere. In this section we'll discuss heavy bleeding that has no apparent cause, often known as "dysfunctional uterine bleeding."

Dysfunctional uterine bleeding often accompanies cycles in which no egg is produced (anovulatory). It's most likely to occur during the early years of your periods and if you are over thirty-five. Though you may bleed heavily, it's not usually especially painful. Serious causes are rare, especially in the first few years of menstruation, and the condition usually settles down by itself in time.

Heavy, irregular bleeding or bleeding that starts after you have completed menopause could be a more serious sign, so you should always see your doctor.

Orthodox treatment

This consists of hormone treatment, the Pill, or drugs that increase the strength of the capillary walls. The problem is that since these don't treat underlying causes your heavy periods will probably return once you stop using the therapy.

D & C (dilatation and curettage), where the lining of the uterus is scraped out, or endometrial aspiration, where it is sucked out, used to be a common treatment for heavy periods. However, these have been shown to have little long-term effect, though they may well be used for purposes of diagnosis. Sometimes, when periods are extremely heavy and don't respond to treatment, hysterectomy is performed. For details of this operation see pages 150, 151.

Alternative therapies and self help

Having ruled out more serious problems, pay close attention to your diet. A lack of vitamin E has been suggested as one cause of heavy periods, and, if you favor nutritional methods, see a nutritionally oriented practitioner. Make sure, too, that you get plenty of green leafy vegetables, wheat germ, liver, parsley, and other iron-rich foods to counteract the possible anemia caused by excessive blood loss.

The stress measures outlined before will help you to relax—meditation and yoga can be especially useful. Both acupuncture and osteopathy have been used in the treatment of menorrhagia.

Herbal remedies that rebalance the hormones are used. David Hoffman, in *The Holistic Herbal* (Findhorn), recommends an infusion of one part American cranesbill, one part beth root, one part periwinkle to be taken three times a day. For further advice consult a qualified herbalist or naturopath.

♫ Menstrual pain (dysmenorrhea)

Menstrual pain can range from mild to severely disabling. How it affects you depends on your individual pain threshold and what else is going on in your life at the time. As always, stress can make it worse.

Doctors have divided menstrual pain into two types: primary dysmenorrhea, which usually starts within a couple of years of beginning to menstruate, and secondary dysmenorrhea, which can begin later in life. In primary dysmenorrhea you experience a low cramp that may spread to your thighs and back, and you may also faint, feel sick or sweaty, or suffer constipation or diarrhea.

Secondary dysmenorrhea tends to start with a general aching in your abdomen about a week to ten days before your period begins, and often goes hand in hand with other premenstrual symptoms. It may stop as soon as your period starts or may last all the way through it. The two types have different causes. Primary is thought to be a result of the uterus contracting, rather as it does when you are in labor, under the influence of prostaglandins. Secondary dysmenorrhea has more wide-ranging causes, which may include pelvic inflammatory disease, endometriosis, fibroids, polyps, or an infection. These are all dealt with elsewhere in this book.

Conventional treatment

For primary dysmenorrhea, regular doses of aspirin, anti-prostaglandin drugs such as ibuprofen (Motrin), or putting you on the Pill are all common. For secondary dysmenorrhea you may be offered antibiotics, hormone treatment, or surgery, depending on the cause.

Self help and alternative treatments

🌊 Hold a covered hot water bottle against your abdomen.

🌊 Take a warm bath or shower.

🌊 Practice relaxation techniques.

🌊 Exercise, especially swimming, dance, or yoga, may all be beneficial. Lying with your legs up against a wall can help relieve that dragging feeling. Ask your yoga teacher to recommend suitable asanas. The cobra is especially useful, as is the bow.

🌊 Visualization is useful when dealing with any sort of pain. Two exercises recommended by Vernon Coleman in *Natural Pain Control* (Century) will help:

1. Imagine your right hand is icy cold. When it feels numb, place it over the painful area and let the numbness soak through.

2. Clasp your right hand as tightly as you can and imagine it is your uterus. Slowly relax it completely. As you do so, your uterus will relax and the pain should gradually ebb away.

It takes a little while to get the hang of using visualization techniques in this way, and you'll need to practice before trying to use them for pain relief.

🌊 Direct massage of the uterus, done by pressing your abdomen just above the pubic hairs and massaging gently, helps the uterus to relax. You may notice that this causes a large clot to be passed, which then relieves pain.

🌊 Herbal treatments include raspberry leaf tea, which you can buy from the health food store. It's an excellent tonic for the uterus. David Hoffmann, in *The Holistic Herbal*, recommends a mixture of two parts black haw bark, two parts cramp bark, and one part pasque flower taken three times a day as an infusion.

🌊 Some self-help homeopathic remedies that may be useful are calcarea carbonica (if you have sore breasts), calcarea phosphorica (if you have a headache), lycopodium (with depression), natrum muriaticum (if you are down and irritable), and pulsatilla (if you are weepy and have painful breasts). If none of these apply, consult a homeopath.

🌊 Acupressure. Direct pressure on the Achilles tendon relieves tension and discomfort.

🌊 Shiatsu massage. Get a friend or your partner to press with the flat of the thumb on either side of the spinal column from your tailbone to your waist: see illustration.

🌊 To relieve constipation, try squeezing half a lemon in some warm water and drink within half an hour of waking up.

🌊 An infusion of ginger—one pinch to a cup of boiling water with honey to taste—during the period is useful.

🌊 Osteopathy can help by freeing blood flow to the pelvis.

🔊 Reflexology is also helpful.

🔊 Acupuncture is especially useful for the treatment of any menstrual problems, possibly because of its endorphin releasing effect.

🔊 TENS (transcutaneous electrical nerve stimulation) is extremely effective for menstrual pain (see page 141).

🔊 Nutritional remedies include a good whole food diet, fasting, and perhaps a supplement of calcium, magnesium, and vitamin D. However, as I've said before, trying to dose yourself with supplements is unwise, so consult a practitioner.

🔊 The following biochemic tissue salts are recommended for painful periods: Mag. Phos., Ferr. Phos., Kali. Phos., Calc. Phos., Kali. Mur., Nat. Mur., Silica.

🔊 Aromatherapy oils include: chamomile, clary sage, cypress, juniper, majoram, lemon, and rosemary.

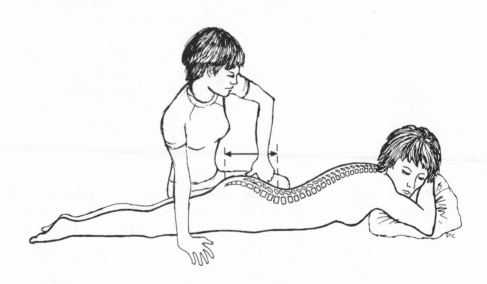

Shiatsu massage for menstrual pain relief.
Lie flat on your stomach and rest your head on a pillow. Get the person applying the massage to press with the flat of the thumb on either side of each of the vertebrae of your spine. Increase pressure slowly, then after a count of ten, ease off.

Fibroids

Fibroids affect about one in five of us over the age of thirty-five. They are non-cancerous lumps that grow in the wall of the uterus. Very often, if the fibroids are small, they cause no trouble at all. But occasionally they can grow much larger—a large fibroid can weigh as much as twenty pounds! In this case they may be responsible for heavy periods, bladder irritation, bleeding between periods, and infertility. Fibroids are dependent on estrogen and usually shrink after menopause.

If the fibroids are small and not causing you any trouble they can usually safely be left alone. In fact, you may not even know you have them unless a doctor comments that you have a "bulky" uterus during an examination. Surgical removal is usually advised for very large fibroids or when you are experiencing a lot of heavy bleeding or pain. Usually, just the fibroid will be removed (myomectomy), which means that you can still have children. But an exceptionally large fibroid may mean a hysterectomy. Is there anything you can do to avoid this?

The answer seems to be a qualified yes.

The first means of treatment for any health problem is always dietary in nature. The best diet for someone attempting to decrease the size of fibroids, or at least keep them from getting any larger, is a whole food semivegetarian diet. Red meat and poultry which may have been fed hormones should not be eaten. Milk products, especially high-fat ones, should also be kept at a minimum.

Since the liver detoxifies excess estrogen, all substances such as alcohol and recreational drugs, which tend to be harmful to the liver, should be eliminated. Coffee and tea should also be kept to a minimum.

If the liver is already sluggish and congested, as it often is in women who develop fibroids, certain herbals such as *Chelidonium* (celandine), *Chionanthus* (fringe tree), or dandelion root may be taken daily to help improve function. It is best to consult a qualified herbalist or naturopath for the proper dosage of these and all liver remedies, as the effects of overstimulation of the liver are unpleasant and may even be dangerous.

Make sure that you drink at least two quarts of water a day during treatment to help your bowels and kidneys work efficiently. What you are trying to do is remove excess estrogen from your system, and this happens more quickly when your organs of elimination are working properly.

Regular exercise is very desirable for anyone attempting to reduce excessive estrogen levels. In fact, some women athletes, especially runners, have reduced their estrogen levels to the point that their periods ceased and they began to

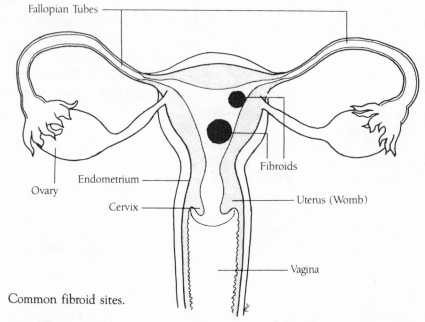

Fallopian Tubes

Endometrium

Ovary

Cervix

Fibroids

Uterus (Womb)

Vagina

Common fibroid sites.

lose bone mass! This, of course, is overdoing it, but it does illustrate how effective exercise can be, especially if you are reducing your ratio of fat to lean body tissue.

Some women have found that the herb *Fraxinus americana* (white ash) has helped reduce the size of their fibroids. Trillium (beth root) has also been useful in helping to control excessive bleeding associated with fibroids. If you are experiencing excessive bleeding, however, you should be closely monitored by your physician, as you could become quite anemic. Heavy bleeding that doesn't respond to less aggressive therapies is a very good reason to have the fibroid surgically removed.

Endometriosis

One of the major causes of heavy, painful periods is endometriosis. It occurs when parts of the lining of the uterus (endometrium) attach themselves to other areas of the pelvis—often the ovaries, fallopian tubes, or the outside of the uterus. The patches of lining grow and bleed with each cycle just as if they were still inside the womb, under the influence of the hormones controlling menstruation. The blood, which is not able to be disposed of in the usual way, forms cysts and scar tissue which causes parts of the pelvic organs to stick together (adhesions). Painful periods, pain between periods, deep pain during intercourse, backache, and infertility are also signs of endometriosis.

☿ Orthodox treatment and diagnosis

A laparoscopy, a procedure that enables the doctor to look at your reproductive organs, will reveal small blood-filled cysts, or larger masses known as "chocolate cysts." Usually treatment consists of stopping hormonal action. Pregnancy can be a temporary respite because of high levels of circulating progesterone. If you want a baby, the doctor may recommend that you become pregnant fairly soon, especially as you could eventually become infertile if the condition worsens.

Orthodox treatment may consist of putting you on a high dose birth control pill, or progesterone type of hormone. A common treatment is the drug danazol (Danocrine), which suppresses the function of the pituitary, the gland controlling the menstrual hormones. In large enough doses, Danocrine can cause the lesions to shrink. The problem is that treatment is expensive and has lengthy and many extremely unpleasant side effects, including weight gain, acne, skin rashes, headaches, muscle cramps, and hairiness. A new nasal contraceptive, which is said to be suitable for treating endometriosis, is at present being tested. It is called Buserelin and works by preventing the pituitary from releasing the luteinizing hormone which is involved in ovulation. Buserelin stops both ovulation and menstruation. But side effects include hot flashes and a dry vagina—the typical menopausal symptoms thought to be caused by low estrogen levels. What's more, the new treatment is unlikely to be available for a few years.

Surgical treatment consists of scraping off the areas affected by endometriosis and freeing any organs trapped by adhesions. If the endometriosis is not widespread and if you want a family, this may be a worthwhile solution. As a last resort you may be offered a hysterectomy and occasionally the removal of your ovaries (oophorectomy). If your ovaries are removed, then you will experience a premature menopause.

☿ Alternative treatment and self help

The key to the proper treatment of endometriosis lies in earlier diagnosis and the prevention of tissue damage, adhesions, and infertility, which cause so much physical pain and heartache. Women often do not realise that persistently painful periods, painful bowel movements, or painful sexual intercourse are very good reasons for visiting their doctors. They may be embarrassed, worry about wasting the doctor's time, or simply disregard these symptoms in the mistaken belief that they are a normal part of being a woman.

Alternative treatment is three-pronged:

___ restoration of health and well-being which has been undermined by months or years of pain and heavy blood loss,

___ soothing pain and alleviating symptoms,

___ restoring hormone balance.

The following *alternative therapies* are recommended:

___ Diet and vitamin therapy. Calcium and magnesium supplements (500 mg of each daily) in the week before your period can alleviate cramps. High doses of vitamin C with added bioflavonoids are said to compensate for high estrogen levels and reduced blood flow. Supplements of A, B, and E vitamins, plus zinc and selenium, are also said to be helpful, as is the ever-versatile evening primrose oil.

___ Biochemic tissue salts.

___ Homeopathy.

___ Herbal medicine. Chaste tree (*Vitex agnus castus*) is a useful treatment since it normalizes the action of the pituitary gland, and especially progesterone production. Wild yam (*Dioscorea villosa*) helps relieve pain and also helps improve progesterone production. Teas such as chamomile, St. John's wort, marigold, lady's mantle, raspberry and hops, fennel and yarrow are recommended. However, since endometriosis is potentially very serious, you are advised to seek the help of a medically qualified herbalist or naturopath and not to try and treat yourself.

___ Acupuncture can ease pain and help normalize the menstrual cycle.

___ Reflexology and aromatherapy may also be used.

___ Yoga may be especially helpful through its relaxing effects, and because it can alter hormone production and restore the nervous system.

___ Nutritional methods—DLPA (phenylalanine) strengthens and protects the body's natural painkillers, endorphins. It's a mixture of two forms of the amino acid (phenylalanine) and is said to be as powerful as morphine, while at the same time being non-addictive and having no side effects. It also seems to help in cases of depression, which is a common feature of endometriosis, as a result of constant pain. You can purchase DLPA at health food stores.

 ♫ Visualization. The following visualization exercise is suggested in the Endometriosis Society leaflet:

"We should think of ways in which we might consciously look after our needs more (as women we have usually been taught that our needs come second) so that we no longer need endometriosis to do that for us. We can consciously use our minds' resources to overcome the illness. We can start by breathing down 'into our stomachs' and relaxing each part of the body in turn from head to toe, and then visualize ourselves in a pleasant natural setting. From there we can move on to visualize the weak, confused endometriosis cells (lost in the wrong place) and the strong purposeful army of white blood cells flooding in with increased blood flow, destroying the endometriosis cells and getting rid of them, soothing pain and tidying up scar tissue. We can visualize our internal organs, pink and healthy, freely mobile, and balanced hormones and see ourselves, healthy and full of energy, achieving the goals we want."

You can do this for a quarter of an hour, about three times a day.

For further information contact:

> The Endometriosis Association
> P.O. Box 92187
> Milwaukee, WI 53202
> Phone: (414) 962-8972

Premenstrual Syndrome

From being virtually unrecognized, premenstrual syndrome (PMS)—or premenstrual tension (PMT) as it is sometimes still called—has received a blast of publicity in both the popular and medical press. It's been estimated that nine out of ten of us may suffer from PMS. But even though PMS is at last receiving serious recognition, confusion as to causes and treatments abounds.

♫ The hormonal clue

What seems certain is that those of us who suffer PMS react in some way to the hormonal changes of the menstrual cycle. But that isn't to say that PMS is *caused* by our hormones. We still don't know the exact relationship between hormones and PMS, nor how diet, pollution, stress, life-style, and personality affect it.

Some experts claim that it's the rise and fall in hormone levels that create PMS. According to this view, estrogen encourages water retention, while prolactin, released by the pituitary under stress, is responsible for breast tenderness. Hormones affect neurotransmitters (chemical messengers) in the brain, especially serotonin, which is responsible for feelings of serenity and tranquility. It's argued that the fall in serotonin levels causes the feelings of anxiety, depression, and so on.

Perhaps the most vociferous promoter of hormonal theories is endocrinologist Katharina Dalton, who believes PMS is caused by progesterone deficiency. However, Dr. Dalton's views are controversial, even among orthodox medics. Endocrine changes can *result* from physical or mental stress rather than being caused by them, and some studies have shown that women with very low concentrations of progesterone do not suffer PMS.

Another theory suggests that prostaglandins produced in the uterus are responsible for the typical cluster of symptoms. However, it's recently been found that cyclical mental and physical symptoms can continue after hysterectomy, neatly refuting that theory.

Yet another theory on the origins of PMS suggests that at certain levels hormones act on the brain, causing a higher level of arousal. Whether you experience this state as positive or negative depends on what else is happening in your life at the time. For instance, if you are under a lot of stress, you will interpret the arousal as negative. If you are feeling loved, supported, and cherished, the time before your period may bring feelings of well-being, increased energy, and elation. This theory makes a lot of sense in view of the many contradictory emotions women with PMS suffer.

⨌ The food connection

Diet seems to play a major role in PMS. Symptoms get worse if you skip meals, and food cravings, especially for sweet things, are common, as is increased appetite. Even orthodox doctors accept that there is a diet connection. In particular, shortages of vitamin B_6, magnesium, iron, and zinc have been implicated. It's known that the Pill, too much coffee and tea, sugar, and alcohol can deplete the body of essential nutrients. Coffee, and smoking in particular, may increase breast tenderness and swelling, as well as affecting mood.

Professor Guy Abrahams, formerly Professor of Obstetrics and Gynecology at the University of California, believes PMS is caused by these three factors:

    ℐ diet,

    ℐ hormone imbalances,

    ℐ stress.

He divides sufferers into four types:

TYPE A: Anxiety, irritability, tension

TYPE B: Bloating, swelling, weight gain

TYPE C: Cravings for sweets, followed by exhaustion, headache, fainting brought about by sudden rise and fall in blood sugar (hypoglycemia)

TYPE D: Depression and confusion

The only catch is that many of us don't fit that easily into any one of these categories; indeed, many women show symptoms of two, three, or all four types.

The following is a table showing the recommended nutrients and amounts needed by women suffering from the various types of PMS.

VITAMIN AND MINERAL SUPPLEMENTATION

Vitamin/Mineral	Dosage*	Comments
Vitamin B-complex	100-400 mg/day	Very helpful in relieving PMS-B and PMS-D.
Calcium	1,000 mg/day, if calcium carbonate is used.	Calcium aspartate and calcium citrate have higher bioavailability and can be used in lower quantities.
Magnesium	1,000-1,500 mg/day	Especially helpful in relieving PMS-C. The old ratio of 2:1 for calcium:magnesium should be reversed. It has been shown that increased calcium intake leads to decreased magnesium absorption. With the current interest in osteoporosis and calcium supplementation, patients with magnesium deficiency are becoming more and more common. To alleviate this, Abraham has shown that the ratio should be reversed. However, too much magnesium leads to diarrhea. It can also result in muscle weakness and sedation. Note that women with impaired kidney function retain magnesium more readily. If calcium intake is high, the ratio should be 2:3 for Ca:Mg. If calcium intake is lower, a 1:2 ratio is better.
Vitamin E	400-600 IU/day	Relieves all types of PMS, especially PMS-B.
Vitamin A	25,000-30,000 IU/day	Relieved headaches in 48 percent of PMS patients in one study.
Zinc	50 mg/day, if zinc glutonate is used	If zinc picolinate is used, less is needed. Especially valuable in relieving PMS-A and PMS-D.
Vitamin C	1,000-1,500 mg/day	Vitamin C competes with estrogen for binding sites on cells and is necessary for the conversion of GLA to PGE.
Gamma linolenic acid (Evening primrose oil)	120-360 mg/day	Especially helpful in relieving PMS-A, PMS-B, and PMS-D.

* *Exact amounts will depend on the severity and type of symptoms, and the patient's diet.*
Source: Holistic Medicine, March-April, 1986. Table prepared by Dr. Kaaren Nichols.

∬ Who gets PMS?

You're more likely to have PMS if:

∬ You are over thirty.

∬ You have two or more children.

∬ Your mother was a PMS sufferer.

∬ You have recently experienced a hormone upheaval—for example, having a baby, coming off the Pill, being sterilized, or if you've been anorexic.

∬ You have had several pregnancies in quick succession.

∬ Treatment

The line between orthodox treatment and alternative treatment is fast becoming blurred. Many PMS clinics offer alternative treatments such as B_6 supplements and evening primrose oil, plus advice on relaxation and so on. Antidepressants and tranquilizers, formerly widely used by conventional doctors, are out after studies showed them to have no value over a placebo. It's probably helpful to think of treatment on a continuum from orthodox to alternative. If you have PMS it's probably a question of finding the right combination of treatment for you.

Main lines of dietary treatment are as follows:

Vitamin B_6

Studies show that a large percentage of PMS sufferers can be helped by supplements of B_6 (pyrodoxine). Some doctors recommend supplements of this and other B complex vitamins, plus magnesium supplements. However, Dr. Katharina Dalton is outspoken in her claim that large supplements of B_6 can cause nervous system symptoms such as tingling or numbness; these disappear once the supplement is stopped. It's probably true to say that megadoses (over 200 mg of B_6 *a day*) should be carried out under the supervision of a nutritionally based practitioner. But smaller doses as outlined below should be safe.

Taking vitamin B_6

∬ Take 50 mg tablets twice a day. You can increase the dose, but don't go above 200 mg a day unless you are under the supervision of a qualified practitioner.

∬ Begin the tablets three days before symptoms usually start and continue until the second or third day of your period, or until the symptoms normally stop. If your periods are irregular it is safe to take the tablets every day.

🗍 Continue for three or four months, then stop to see whether they have helped. If they have, you can safely continue.

🗍 If the method doesn't work, or if you experience side effects such as numbness or tingling, stop the treatment and consult your doctor or an alternative practitioner.

🗍 If you get pregnant, stop taking the supplement, as there is a suggestion that large amounts might cause birth defects.

Evening primrose oil

Studies have long suggested that women with PMS can be helped by taking evening primrose oil. It's especially useful if you suffer breast discomfort, eczema, irritability or depression, or if you are diabetic.

Evening primrose oil is thought to work because it is rich in a rare essential fatty acid (gammalinolenic acid, or GLA for short) that converts into prostaglandin E in the body. A diet too rich in animal fats, processed oils, and alcohol, as well as certain viruses, cancer, and exposure to radiation, all affect the body's ability to form GLA, and may explain why many women are short of it.

Side effects are uncommon, but some women experience diarrhea or stomach upsets, and a few are allergic to the gelatin which is used in the capsule, in which case you can get drops.

Take two 500 mg capsules twice a day after food, starting three days before symptoms usually start. You may need more or less, depending on how you respond, and advice on this can be found in *The Premenstrual Syndrome* by Dr. Caroline Shreeve (Thorsons). Evening primrose oil is made more effective if you take it with a vitamin and mineral supplement which contains vitamin B_6, vitamin C, and zinc.

Does it work?

These are some of the comments made in a *Here's Health* study of the effectiveness of evening primrose oil:

"Stomach cramps and bloated stomach disappeared."

"Premenstrual symptoms greatly reduced in first month and almost disappeared in second."

"Dramatic effect. No monthly 'row' with husband."

"Period pain reduced from severe to absent. Will buy if I can afford."

Other supplements

Vitamin E can help some women with PMS (take 150-600 IU a day). Magnesium supplements are also helpful for most women.

What you eat

Observe the following good food rules:

⊿ Eat whole grains, nuts, and seeds. Almonds, coconut, sesame, and sunflower seeds provide potassium, which may be depleted if you have PMS.

⊿ Avoid tea, coffee, cocoa, coke-type drinks, and alcohol. Substitute spring water and herb teas.

⊿ Eat small, frequent meals to dispel sugar cravings and keep up blood sugar levels.

⊿ Include plenty of raw foods in what you eat.

⊿ Limit dairy foods, as they may interfere with magnesium absorption. Good sources of magnesium include green leafy vegetables and lentils.

⊿ Cut out junk foods, sweets, cakes, and pastries: they can cause water retention and prevent the body from absorbing essential minerals.

⊿ Cut salt intake if bloating is a problem.

Hormone treatments

These may include the Pill—although many doctors think that this actually aggravates symptoms—and artifical and natural hormones of the progesterone family. However, side effects can be troublesome, including breast tenderness, headaches, varicose veins, hemorrhoids, and vaginal infections. Dr. Katharina Dalton argues that only pure progesterone in the form of suppositories or injections should be used. But many doctors disagree, and progesterone can cause unwelcome side effects.

Danocrine, which is described in the section on endometriosis, may also be prescribed, though for many women the side effects are worse than the PMS.

Estradiol implants

The newest and most controversial treatment aims to suppress ovulation in an attempt to control hormonal fluctuations. It involves injecting implants of estradiol, a type of estrogen, under the skin of your stomach. Many orthodox doctors violently oppose the treatment. It can cause menstrual irregularities and other problems which may be very hard to deal with once the implant is there.

Nonhormone drug therapies

These include antiprostaglandins, such as mefanamic acid (Ponstel), and bromocriptine, which reduces prolactin production. However, bromocriptine can cause vomiting and some doctors believe it is dangerous. The use of diuretics to get rid of swelling is also recommended by some doctors, although others argue that this doesn't really treat the root of PMS and only deals with a symptom. What's more, some diuretics can deplete the body of potassium.

Herbal remedies

There are numerous herbal treatments for PMS. Scullcap and valerian in tablet form can ease tension. Dandelion, though bitter, can help with fluid retention. One of the best herbal treatments is *Vitex agnus castus* (chaste tree), a progesteronelike herb that helps improve pituitary function and balance hormone levels.

Dioscorea (wild yam) is also a very effective herbal in the treatment of PMS. Its action is similar to that of *Vitex agnus castus*. Go to a qualified herbal practitioner or naturopath for all but the simplest treatments.

Homeopathic treatment

This is often very successful. The following self-help remedies have been suggested: calcaria carbonica, (with tender breasts), graphites (with weight gain), lycopodium (with depression), natrum muriaticum (with irritability), nux vomica (if you are argumentative), pulsatilla (if you are weepy), and sepia (if you suffer mood swings). You are advised to consult a qualified homeopath, who will look at you as a whole and try to find the best remedy for you as a person.

Acupuncture and acupressure

Both see PMS as a result of imbalance or blockage of vital energy or chi, and there are many excellent results reported from using them.

Osteopathy, reflexology, and aromatherapy can all help too.

Other factors to consider

Smoking

Recent studies show that smoking interferes with blood flow, and increases the secretion of stress hormones. Evening primrose oil was shown to improve blood flow in smokers. Better still—try and give up altogther!

Stress

Stress can deplete magnesium in the body, so follow the stress-relieving tips outlined earlier. Yoga, meditation, T'ai Chi, and dance are just some of the therapies that may be useful.

A menstrual diary

Keep a diary for three to four months, either on the lines of the one illustrated, or a written record if you find that easier. Note mood changes and physical symptoms. Record feelings of well-being and energy, as well as more negative feelings. It's all too easy to record a bout of irritability coming before a period, but dismiss such a mood as unimportant afterward. What you're aiming for is an *awareness* of mood fluctuations over the whole of your cycle.

Managing your moods

Once you've got a picture of your mood changes, you can start to deal with them. PMS may alert you to issues in your life that need attention. The feelings of frustration, anger, hopelessness, and so on that many of us feel premenstrually aren't entirely negative. They can be valuable pointers to areas of your life that need tackling.

Of course there may be some problems you can't do anything about. You may, for example, be struggling to manage on too little money, or be feeling isolated or overwhelmed by the demands of young children. But that doesn't mean these problems don't matter. Women often feel it's wrong or "unfeminine" to be angry. Accepting your right to be angry or depressed may help you feel less stressed. Seeing that a problem that you thought just affected you is more widespread may prompt you to join a group working for wider change.

On a more personal level, dealing with your emotions might include psychotherapy to help you identify and deal with problems that upset you premenstrually, counseling, or assertiveness training to help you cope with anger more constructively.

Try to make life easy for yourself in the time before your period. Save heavy jobs around the house, difficult meetings at work, and awkward discussions until after your period, if you can. Meditation, a warm bath, a walk, talking to a friend, painting, sex (with a partner or by masturbation) can all help release tension and help you to relax.

MONTH ⟶

DAY	1	2	3	4	5	6	7	8	9	10	11	12
1												
2												
3												
4												
5												
6												
7												
8												
9												
10												
11												
12												
13												
14												
15												
16												
17												
18												
19												
20												
21												
22												
23												
24												
25												
26												
27												
28												
29												
30												
31												

Example of a menstrual diary.

Indicate each day of your menstruation with an 'M' or other such mark in the appropriate square.

Indicate each day on which you experience the following symptoms by using the letters from this key:

D—Depression
P—Pain (backache or headache)
F—Fatigue

T—Tension, Irritability, or Anxiety
BT—Breast Tenderness
B—Bloated Feeling

Support and help

Enlist the help of friends and family at this time. Join a PMS support group, or seek out a special PMS clinic or alternative practitioner.

The National Women's Health Network, 224 7th St. NE, Washington, DC 20003, should have information about groups near you.

☞ Headaches and migraine

Migraine affects one in five of us and is more common in women than in men. If you suffer headaches or migraine you are most likely to have them in the week leading up to your period. The highest incidence of headaches and migraine is found in those on the Pill. There are a number of triggers for an attack, which include:

☞ Alcohol.

☞ Fried or fatty food, pork, pickled herring.

☞ Skipping meals.

☞ Certain types of food—commonly chocolate, cheese and dairy products, citrus fruits, vegetables, tea and coffee, meat, seafood.

That's not to say that food is the sole reason for all migraine attacks; some people simply seem to be born with a tendency toward it.

Tension headaches are often brought on by physical or mental stress, for example, driving a car with your head held in the same position for a long time.

Research is currently being carried out at St. Thomas Hospital, London, to see whether there is a hormone connection between certain types of headache and migraine. In the meantime, the following self-help and alternative methods may help.

☞ Keep a diary so that you can see if there is a pattern to the headaches.

☞ Don't skip meals, especially breakfast.

☞ Try to get a "proper" meal at lunchtime.

☞ Eat regularly. If you're going out in the evening, try to have something to eat before you go.

☞ If you develop an attack, try to eat something, as lack of food makes it worse.

☞ Niacin at the beginning of an attack—100 mg every fifteen minutes until flushing occurs—helps many people.

☞ Acupuncture or acupressure.

☞ Reflexology.

☞ Therapeutic touch (laying on of hands).

𝒥 Herbal medicine, especially the ancient herbal remedy feverfew, has recently received the thumbs up sign from conventional medicine. You can either eat feverfew in a sandwich or make it into a tea, or get it in tablet form from the health food store.

𝒥 Homeopathic dosages of feverfew are now available, and there are a number of other homeopathic remedies helpful for those who suffer migraines.

𝒥 Biochemic tissue salts.

𝒥 Yoga has a number of useful postures.

𝒥 Meditation and relaxation.

𝒥 Dealing with anger

It can be good sometimes to let off steam, but often, especially if you have PMS, anger can appear to be controlling you. Learning how to manage your anger can give you greater control over a situation.

STEP ONE: Identify situations that make you angry and work out exactly what it is that annoys you, and how you normally deal with it.

STEP TWO: Involves what an anger control expert—yes, there really is such a thing—calls "changing your inner dialogue." In other words, you talk yourself through difficult confrontations.

Ready ...

Say to yourself: "I know that this is going to make me angry, but I know how to deal with it. I can use my energy to manage this situation , and keep my sense of humor". It may feel a little artifical at first, but you'll soon get used to it and be able to think of statements of your own.

... Steady ...

As you go into the confrontation, remind yourself:

"I am going to stay calm. There's no point in building a mountain out of a molehill. I can cope."

... Go

While you're doing this, continue to monitor how you feel:

"I can feel my muscles getting tense. Relax. Take it step by step."

STEP THREE: Once the confrontation is over, think positively about the incident:

"It's all over now, I can forget about it. I didn't do too badly that time. Next time I'll do even better." Don't blame yourself if you did lose your cool. Breathe deeply and resolve to try again next time. If you did manage to cope with the situation, congratulate yourself—you deserve it!

Do you suffer from PMS?

Over 150 symptoms have been listed by PMS sufferers.

How many of them apply to you?

☐ Feelings of depression, sadness, pessimism.

☐ Tiredness, lethargy, feelings of being "under the weather."

☐ Tension, irritability, anxiety.

☐ Increased or decreased appetite.

☐ Craving for sweet or salty foods.

☐ Thirst.

☐ Lack of concentration, difficulties in decision-making.

☐ Weepiness.

☐ Mood swings.

☐ Feeling extra sexy or losing interest in sex.

☐ Inability to sleep or wanting to sleep all the time.

☐ Aggressive outbursts, impulsive behavior.

☐ Increased energy.

☐ Loss of confidence and self-esteem, wanting to stay indoors all the time.

☐ Guilt feelings, putting yourself down.

☐ Loss of interest in yourself.

☐ Apathy.

☐ Headache or migraine.

☐ Breast swelling and tenderness.

☐ Bloating or feeling of bloatedness.

☐ Swollen fingers and toes.

☐ Acne, rashes, itching.

☐ Constipation, nausea, diarrhea.

☐ Poor coordination, clumsiness, becoming "accident-prone."

☐ Muscle weakness, backache, muscle pain.

☐ Dizziness.

☐ Weight gain.

☐ Increased sweatiness.

☐ Blurred vision, sore eyes.

☐ Passing an increased or decreased amount of urine.

☐ Pain low in the abdomen.

☐ Increased vaginal discharge.

☐ Decreased efficiency.

Based on *The Premenstrual Syndrome* by Maurice Katz (Update Postgraduate Centre Series, Update Publications, 1984).

Vaginal Infections

The vagina is self-cleansing, and all of us secrete mucus made up of cells from the vagina and cervix. At certain times in our lives—for instance, in our teens, during pregnancy, at certain times during the menstrual cycle, during sexual arousal, and on the Pill, the discharge can increase. A normal vaginal discharge is clear and sticky, whitish-yellow, or white and creamy, depending on the stage of your menstrual cycle. Daily washing of your genital area is sufficient to keep clean under most normal conditions, and there's no need to wash inside your vagina itself. However, if the discharge becomes different in color or texture, and especially if the amount is more than usual or changes in smell, you could have an infection. This section gives a rundown of the causes of vaginal discharge, noninfectious and infectious varieties, and the orthodox and alternative treatments.

Once the cause of the discharge is removed, the symptoms will disappear of their own accord (see "Preventing vaginal infections"—page 71)

Noninfectious causes of vaginal discharge:

- If you are just starting your periods
- Various times during your menstrual cycle
- When you are sexually active
- During pregnancy
- During menopause
- A forgotten tampon or other foreign body in the vagina
- Chemicals such as bubble baths, soap, or douches
- Drug-related discharge, e.g., if you are on the Pill, have been taking antibiotics, or use contraceptive inserts or gel
- Certain gynecological problems such as cervical erosion

Infectious causes of vaginal discharge:

- Yeast (Monilia)
- Trichomonas (Trich)
- Bacterial infection (anerobic, vaginitis, e.g., gardenerella)
- Chlamydia
- Herpes
- Gonorrhea

Yeast (Monilia)

Yeast is caused by a fungal organism (*Candida albicans*) that normally lives in places such as the vagina, anus, and under the fingernails, without causing any trouble. The fungus thrives in a high sugar environment, so that if the normally slightly acid environment of the vagina is disturbed in any way it goes out of control. Times when this may occur are if you have a high intake of sugar in your diet, if you have diabetes, during pregnancy and during the second half of your menstrual cycle, or if you are on a high-dose Pill. Some men's semen appears to be more alkaline than others, which may trigger an attack, especially if you have a new partner. A man with yeast can transmit it to you even if he has no symptoms himself. If you are run-down or under stress, an attack may be triggered if you are susceptible. A course of antibiotic treatment, by killing the bacteria that normally keep *Candida* in balance, often creates just the right conditions for yeast to grow.

Classic symptoms of a *candida* infection are a white cheesy discharge that smells yeasty, buring on urination, and extreme soreness and itchiness of the whole vulva. There is often visible inflammation, which may spread to the inner thighs. Less severe but still bothersome infections may have a scanty serous discharge and less visible inflammation but still have soreness and itching.

Orthodox diagnosis and treatment

The doctor will examine you—this may be sufficient to diagnose a yeast infection. The doctor may also want to take a swab to be analyzed in the lab to rule out any other infections, and may also carry out a simple pH (acid-alkaline) test, using color-sensitive paper to confirm whether the discharge is acid or alkaline. Treatment is with suppositories, cream, and/or tablets (Mycostatin and Mycolog being the most commonly used), and sometimes a special jelly to correct acid balance in the vagina. Occasionally, where itchiness is extremely severe, you may be given gentian violet. This is extremely soothing but beware— it's horribly messy!

Unfortunately, yeast has a nasty habit of coming back unless you tackle the root causes, such as diet, stress, or an unhealthy life-style. Women who suffer from recurrent yeast often feel thoroughly miserable and "unclean". Recurrent yeast infections continue to defy orthodox treatment, and the best your doctor will be able to do in many cases is to suggest long-term nystatin treatment. Many of us dislike the thought of being on medication virtually indefinitely, so what else can you do?

Self help and alternative therapies

The answer is a combination of self help and alternative treatment. The connection between recurrent yeast and stress, plus other facets of life-style, is crucial from the alternative viewpoint. Following the preventive tips outlined here will help decrease your chances of developing an attack. At the first signs of a yeast infection:

✍ Treat it with the most effective home treatment for most women, the vaginal insertion of boric acid and acidophilus capsules. Fill 00 capsules with boric acid powder, available at any drugstore, and use one capsule of this and two capsules of acidophilus inserted high into the vagina every night for five to seven nights. Some women find the boric acid too harsh; if you experience more than slight discomfort with this method, douche to remove the boric acid and use one of the milder remedies. Also, you should not use this method if you are pregnant. In any case, do not use boric acid more than seven nights in a row or more often than once a month without a doctor's permission.

✍ Add salt to your bath—enough to make the water taste slightly salty.

✍ Use a vinegar and water douche—1 tablespoon vinegar to 1 pint water—twice a day for a day or so to help rebalance the vaginal environment. Alternatively, soak a tampon in the same quantities of solution and insert into your vagina. Never use straight vinegar because it will sting.

✍ Apply natural, unsweetened live yogurt, using a tampon, applicator, plastic syringe, or speculum. This is a slow but sure method—it takes some ten to fifteen days. Note, though, that some doctors have warned against this practice on the grounds that it can cause pregnancy complications. In any case, you should never put anything in your vagina if you think you might be pregnant.

✍ Herbal remedies for yeast infections include compresses of golden seal, comfrey, crab apples, bay bark, myrrh, or thuja ointment from the health food store or an herbal supplier. Unless you are familiar with herbs and their uses, consult a qualified herbalist or naturopath, as all these remedies are expensive.

✍ Some practitioners recommend inserting a clove of garlic wrapped in cheesecloth into your vagina. However, some women have complained that this stings. Try it—but if it's too uncomfortable don't continue.

✍ Avoid sex with penetration until the yeast has cleared up.

Diet

A sugary diet, as we've already said, can predispose to yeast. Eat a good whole food diet, and cut out alcohol and any foods containing mold or fungus, such as Stilton cheese, mushrooms, and so on. On a naturopathic regimen you'll be advised to stay off fruit because of its high sugar content, and to take a supplement of *Lactobacillus acidophilus*—a bacterium which is killed by antibiotics. Vitamin B and C supplements may also be advised. Some experts recommend eating live yogurt, as well as applying it directly.

Homeopathy

Homeopathy has many useful remedies for vaginal discharge. A pilot study carried out in 1984 in orthodox clinics showed that a combination of two homeopathic remedies, borax and candida, was significantly more effective than a placebo in treating certain women with yeast infections. It's not advised that you try to treat yourself with these, however, since they might not be indicated in your case.

The yeast connection

Some clinical ecologists (see page 160) go one step farther and blame *Candida albicans* (the organism involved in yeast) for being behind a whole host of other, seemingly unconnected ailments. These include diseases as apparently diverse as AIDS, multiple sclerosis, migraine, schizophrenia, PMS, and arthritis. An article in the journal *Healthsharing*, Summer 1985, states: "It's estimated that 30 percent of the population is susceptible to severe candida infections. Women are affected more often than men." The article blames modern life-styles: antibiotics, the Pill, diet, chemicals at work, and stress-related hormone imbalances for the epidemic of yeast-related diseases.

According to this view, such factors weaken the immune system, leaving the body open for candida invasion. The way it affects you will depend on a number of factors, including genetic susceptibility.

Advice consists of putting you on a diet low in sugary and starchy foods, as well as dried herbs and teas and pickled and smoked foods. This suggested diet is commonly supplemented with some sort of antifungal, such as nystatin, to kill the yeast, and a high-potency acidophilus preparation to help rebalance bowel flora and increase resistance to infection.

It has to be said that this approach is highly controversial and most orthodox doctors would dismiss it entirely. As always, in the absence of controlled trials, it's difficult to be certain. But if you do suffer from recurrent yeast for which no other treatment seems to work, it may well be worth consulting a clinical ecologist or other allergy specialist.

For further information:

The Yeast Connection, Dr. William Crook (Professional Books).

The Missing Diagnosis. Dr. C.O. Truss (Missing Diagnosis, Inc.)

Candida Albicans, Leon Chaitow, N.D. (Thorsons)

☞ Trich or TV *(Trichomonas vaginalis)*

Trich is caused by a one-celled organism, which, like *Candida*, is often already present in the vagina, anus, cervix, urethra, or bladder, where it normally doesn't present problems. The discharge is frothy and is yellowish-green with an unpleasant smell. You will be red and sore, and have a burning sensation when you urinate. Your cervix may be inflamed "like a strawberry." Trich is usually sexually transmitted, but you can catch it from other sources since it lives for several hours at room temperature in a moist atmosphere. For instance, you could catch it from a wet swimsuit, toilet seat, towel, or washcloth that has been used by someone with trich.

The infection often occurs with other sexually transmitted infections such as gonorrhea. There's a great chance that your sex partner will be infected too, so both of you should be treated even if he or she has no apparent symptoms.

It may be worse immediately after or before your period because of the altered pH level in your vagina at this time. Like yeast, trich is more likely to take hold if you are already run down.

☞ Bacterial vaginal infections (nonspecific vaginitis)

Nonspecific vaginitis is an umbrella term used by doctors to describe a variety of bacterial infections. The most common sort is perhaps gardenrella *(Corynebacterium vaginalis)*. Symptoms are a thin, watery, fishy-smelling discharge. The smell often gets worse mid-cycle or after sex. Your partner may be infected too, but have no symptoms.

Orthodox treatment

Flagyl (metronidazole), a very powerful antibiotic, is the first line of treatment for both these infections. Alternatively, for nonspecific vaginitis other antibiotics are sometimes used, although these may be less effective and may lead to yeast infections. Flagyl is an extremely powerful drug, and it's important that you not take it during the first three months of pregnancy. It can have side effects such as nausea, stomach upsets, and headaches, and can also affect your white blood cell production. For this reason, your doctor may want to take blood tests to see how you are responding to the drug. Flagyl also reacts with alcohol, so you should cut out drinking.

♂ Chlamydia

This is a fairly recently discovered viruslike organism.

Younger women and those on the Pill are especially at risk. If left untreated it can lead to pelvic inflammatory disease (PID), a major cause of infertility.

There may be no symptoms initially, or you may feel like you have a bladder infection. Later symptoms include a raised temperature, pain on moving your bowels, and a pus or blood-stained discharge. Your cervix is inflamed, and there may be deep pelvic pain. If chlamydia is passed on to your unborn baby it can cause eye infection after birth, breathing difficulties, and very occasionally even blindness.

The main problem with chlamydia is that it is often symptomless. If you have any reason to suspect that your partner may have an infection, it's worth going for a test to your nearest health clinic. Treatment is with powerful antibiotics such as Flagyl, tetracycline, or erythromycin. Tetracycline shouldn't be used if you are pregnant, as it can stain your baby's teeth yellow.

♂ Gonorrhea and syphilis

These two used to be the most common venereal diseases, although these days chlamydia and herpes are more common. Of the two, gonorrhea is the most common and may be especially difficult to treat because it is often symptomless in women. If left untreated it's a major cause of blocked tubes leading to sterility. It often goes hand in hand with chlamydia, and if you have one you should always be tested for the other, since just treating the gonorrhea may mask the chlamydia with the subsequent risk of developing pelvic inflammatory disease. Where symptoms do appear, they develop within five to seven days of sexual contact. You'll have an offensive yellow discharge, pain when you urinate, and frequency of urination.

Syphilis is rarer and even harder to detect. It has an incubation period of between two weeks and a month, and sometimes even longer. It's much more common in men than in women. If left untreated it can eventually lead to diseases of the heart and nervous system. Symptoms start with a small painless sore that, left untreated, heals within six to ten weeks. You may get swollen glands in the groin, or have other swollen lymph glands. Treatment of both syphilis and gonorrhea is with large doses of antibiotics, and if carried out at an early stage it is usually 100 percent successful.

♫ Alternative medicine and self help

The only acceptable treatment of gonorrhea, syphilis, and chlamydia is by antibiotics. However, there are plenty of other steps you can take to improve your resistance so that your body can fight off these infections more effectively. What's more, alternative treatments can provide a useful back-up to conventional treatment. An orthodox doctor who is also qualified in alternative therapies can, of course, treat you. Homeopathy in particular has some useful remedies. An herbalist may advise douches and compresses, for instance, of golden seal, myrrh, or comfrey to mention a few. Aromatherapy oils can be useful either taken by mouth or in a sitz bath, and can help increase the effectiveness of antibiotics. But all of these are probably best used as an adjunct to conventional treatment rather than a first line of defense.

♫ Preventing vaginal infections

If you practice self-examination as described in Part One, you may be able to spot an incipient infection before it gets a chance to take hold, so you can immediately put a preventive plan into action.

♫ Pay attention to diet. In particular cut down on sugary foods. A drink of a teaspoon of honey and vinegar in hot water will help maintain the vagina's normally slightly acid environment.

♫ Get plenty of rest and sleep.

♫ If you are run down or under stress, follow the stress management strategies outlined elsewhere. Meditation, yoga, T'ai Chi, or any of the mind-body therapies may be helpful.

♫ Avoid reusing washcloths to wash the genital area, as these can harbor germs.

♫ Always wipe from front to back after moving your bowels to prevent contamination of the vagina with bacteria from the anus.

♫ Avoid vaginal deodorant sprays, talc, scented soap, and bubble or antiseptic bath solutions.

♫ Use cotton underwear.

♫ Avoid tight pants. Expose the area to air and sunlight if you get the opportunity!

♫ Take your swimsuit off immediately

after you get out of the water and allow it to dry.

⚐ Keep your nails short and your hands clean.

⚐ A cupful of vinegar in the bath water occasionally will help maintain the acid balance of your vagina.

⚐ Make sure your partner keeps his penis and beneath the foreskin clean.

⚐ Avoid colored toilet paper.

⚐ Practice pelvic floor exercises as described in Part One to increase circulation to the area.

⚐ For relief of itching, apply a compress of live culture yogurt several times a day. Alternatively, bathe your genitals in a sage or chickweed infusion. For further details of herbal douches and compresses for vaginal infections, see *The Holistic Herbal* by David Hoffman (Findhorn).

⚐ Herpes

So far we've looked at bacterial infections. More difficult to treat are virus infections. The main one is herpes, or herpes simplex to give it its full name.

Genital herpes, or herpes 2, is a form of the virus herpes that causes cold sores around the mouth, and is now the second most common sexually transmitted disease, especially in women. So far there is no permanent cure, although there are many ways you can help keep herpes at bay or shorten an attack should you develop one.

On the whole, herpes is more a nuisance than it is dangerous, except that there is an as yet unproven suggestion that cervical cancer may be more common if you have herpes. Herpes can also be passed on to your unborn baby if you are pregnant. If this happens, it can be very serious or even fatal to your baby. If you have clinical or laboratory evidence of herpes at the time of birth, you'll be advised to have a caesarean.

Herpes is often picked up through sexual contact, although not always. It may be transferred from mouth to genitals during oral sex, via the fingers, or even on damp towels or washcloths. The point to bear in mind is that you must have had some sort of contact with an open herpes sore. At this stage you will develop a first infection between two and twenty days after exposure. The commonest time is about a week after contact. The first attack of herpes is usually the worst. The first sign is a tingling or burning sensation, followed by fluid-filled sores which burst to form ulcers, which then scab over and heal. You may develop swollen, tender glands in your groin, a fever, a headache, and a general fluish feeling. The infection may last for up to three weeks. Subsequent infections aren't usually so severe or long lasting. But once you have developed the sores the virus remains in your body, where it can be reactivated, often if you are run down or under stress. Other triggers include having another illness which produces a high fever, exposure to ultraviolet light (e.g., when you sunbathe,) menstruation, or injury.

You are contagious from the time you feel the signs until the sores have healed over completely.

Orthodox treatment

See your doctor as soon as the first symptoms appear so that a swab test can be made. This is important to rule out the possibility of other STDs and to confirm the diagnosis.

Orthodox treatment is limited at the moment. It consists of anesthetic gels or ointments to relieve pain, plus painkillers such as aspirin or something stronger to be taken by mouth. You'll usually be given an anesthetic jelly such as Xylocaine to smooth on before urinating, to reduce burning and stinging. You may also be given antibiotics to prevent or treat any secondary bacterial infection you may have picked up. There are also a number of antiviral drugs now available. The main trouble with these in the past has been that they killed not only the virus but the cell along with it, so causing a number of unpleasant side effects. The most promising new development is a drug called acyclovir (Zovirax), which seems, according to the doctor's journal *The Practitionery*, to be "remarkably free of side effects." It appears to be effective in cutting short the length of the attack as well as the time it takes for the sores to heal.

There are also reports of a new vaccine, not yet available, which may help prevent recurrent attacks.

But acyclovir can't prevent future attacks. It's only fair to say that many people experience just one episode of herpes and that's it. But some will go on to develop further attacks, especially when run down or under stress.

So what does alternative medicine have to offer?

Self help and alternative therapies

The alternative approach focuses on diet. Two amino acids, arginine and lysine, have been found to play a big part in preventing or encouraging attacks of herpes. A diet high in lysine (found in foods such as fresh fish, chicken, cheese, lima beans, cottage cheese, beansprouts, and prawns) has been found to inhibit attacks. A diet high in arginine (found in various types of nuts, sesame seeds, cocoa, brown rice, whole-grain bread, raisins, and sunflower seeds) has been found to promote an outbreak. It's important to grasp the fact that these foods don't cause herpes, but they may predispose you to an attack if you already have the virus in a dormant form.

Some naturopaths claim complete remission of the disease, but you have to follow treatment to the letter for it to be effective. Extra A, B, C, and E vitamins may help prevent attacks.

High lysine foods: fish, chicken, beef, milk, lamb, pork, lima beans, cottage cheese, mung beansprouts, shrimp, prawns, soybeans, eggs.

High arginine foods: hazelnuts, brazil nuts, peanuts, walnuts, almonds, cocoa, peanut butter, sesame seeds, cashew nuts, carob powder, coconut, pistachio nuts, buckwheat flour, chick peas, brown rice, pecans, whole grain bread, cooked oatmeal, raisins, sunflower seeds.

The immune system

Your immune system is the other mainstay of any alternative approach to herpes. As North and Crittenden say in *Stop Herpes Now!* (Thorsons): "A healthy immune system can keep the virus quietly under control...help your body resist infection from herpes—use good nutrition, exercise and conscious stress-reduction techniques to keep your immune system in top condition."

Alternative techniques such as meditation, which can sometimes have a direct effect on the immune system, hypnosis, yoga, (visualization techniques), and relaxation can all help. Other therapies which have helped some people include homeopathy, acupuncture, and herbalism. The best herbals for use in treating herpes are echinacea, thuja, and golden seal internally to help support the immune system. Certain licorice root preparations are useful locally. One of the best is called Herplic. It is available through many naturopaths and some herbalists.

For relief of herpes

✍ Enjoy a warm bath or a sitz bath with salt added to relieve discomfort.

✍ Apply ice packs to the affected area.

✍ Wear cotton underwear.

✍ Keep the sores clean and dry. Wash with soap and water.

✍ Cold tea bags can reduce inflammation.

✍ Pay attention to diet. Eat foods high in lysine and low in arginine.

To prevent attacks

✐ Learn what triggers an attack. Keeping a diary will help.

✐ Eat a diet high in raw foods and low in fat and sugar. Continue to eat high lysine foods or take lysine tablets, available from the health food store.

✐ Avoid or deal with unnecessary stress.

✐ See a nutritionally qualified practitioner and find out if mineral supplements would benefit you.

✐ Visit a holistic G.P. or naturopath to find out about dietary changes you could make.

✐ See a medically qualified homeopath. There are a number of homeopathic remedies which may help.

To avoid herpes

✐ Don't touch cold sores around the mouth or genitals of a partner or friend.

✐ Don't share washcloths, sponges, towels, lipstick, or other intimate items with anyone else.

✐ If you have a new partner, find out whether he or she has ever had herpes.

✐ Use condoms for safety.

✐ Don't have sex with penetration or masturbation when open sores are present.

✐ Pay attention to diet, exercise, and stress management.

You and your partner

If you've had herpes in the past, you may feel depressed and anxious, and as though you have no right to have sex. It's only fair to warn a new partner if you have had herpes. Open, honest discussion of the risks of infection and how you can deal with the problem together will go a long way toward helping you deal with it. A Herpes Association pamphlet "Herpes simplex and You" stresses, "Herpes is not you. You just have a rash which occasionally gets in the way. When you can handle the contagion problem, the emotional concerns will diminish." Of course, you can't entirely rule out the possibility of infecting your partner, but with sensible measures of the sort outlined above, you can reduce the risks to the minimum. Even if intercourse, masturbation, or oral sex is out, there are plenty of other ways you can enjoy each other sexually. Now is your chance to be creative and find out new ways to please each other.

♫ Genital warts

These are caused by a virus which is usually passed on sexually. They don't hurt, but they may itch or bleed. Vigorous sex or wearing tight-fitting jeans can irritate them, and they thrive in a warm, moist atmosphere. Genital warts (human papillomavirus, or HPV) are an increasing problem. Until recently they were considered only a minor nuisance, however, recent studies have suggested a strong connection between HPV virus and the subsequent development of cancer of the cervix.

As with herpes there's no way of preventing recurrence. Conventional treatment consists of burning them off or using a caustic resin called podophyllum.

If you've had genital warts, you should make sure you go for regular Pap tests so that any early signs of cervical cancer can be treated at an early stage.

Alternative treatments

There's little information available on alternative treatments. However, thuja ointment or tincture can be used, either by an herbalist or in homeopathic doses. Acupuncture and homeopathy can both help tone up the system so your body can resist the infection more readily.

Other Vaginal Problems

♫ Cervical erosion

When cells from inside the cervix (the neck of the womb) spread to the outside, a red, shiny area develops that may produce increased mucus. Sometimes the erosion may become infected.

Erosion occurs because of an excess of estrogen. That means you are more likely to develop one if you are pregnant, on the Pill, or at other times of hormonal upset, for instance, if you are under stress.

Occasionally, an erosion may bleed after sex, but it's usually painless, and you may not even know you have one unless the doctor mentions it when you have an internal exam or you see it yourself during self-examination.

Usually an uninfected erosion is best left alone, since if treatment merely removes the erosion without treating any underlying hormone imbalance, it will only come back. However, if the discharge becomes troublesome or you develop a tendency to cervicitis or vaginal infections, you should seek treatment. Conventional treatment consists of burning or freezing off the cells. This is not nearly as gruesome as it sounds.

Alternative treatments and self help

Alternative therapies which treat underlying imbalances are especially useful. Acupuncture, for example, helps "tune up" the body and removes imbalances. Herbal remedies can be very useful. Golden seal is, according to one medical herbalist, "a marvelous treatment, but it stains everything yellow, and is expensive." You'd be advised to consult a qualified herbalist or naturopath rather than trying to treat yourself. Homeopathic remedies are also useful. Cold sitz baths and practicing your pelvic floor exercises will increase circulation to the area.

Many naturopaths use a series of herbal drawing packs, along with diet and nutritional therapies, to heal infected erosions. This treatment, over time, also slowly causes regression of the erosion itself. Any treatment which helps reduce stress, for example, meditation, yoga, relaxation techniques, and so on is worthwhile, as stress can upset your hormones (see section on menstrual periods, page 43).

ℐ Bartholin gland cysts and abscesses

The Bartholin glands are two small, rounded glands that lie on either side of your vagina and produce mucus when you get sexually aroused. Occasionally, one or both of the ducts that normally drain away these secretions become blocked and a cyst develops. Conventional treatment ususally consists of doing nothing or, if the blocked gland becomes troublesome, lancing it to release the fluid, inserting a drain, and applying antibiotic cream or ointment.

It is not unusual for gonorrhea to cause an infection of the Bartholin gland, so if you are having a problem this should be checked.

If you have a gland which is frequently infected or is causing you problems because of its size, your doctor may suggest an operation which basically gives the gland a new outlet. It's called *marsupialization* and is generally successful in solving the problem.

Alternative treatments

Hot and cold sitz baths to increase circulation and stimulate glandular activity or hot and cold compresses may be used. An herbalist may recommend a local ointment or lotion, or a solution of goosegrass or cleavers. Golden seal, again, reduces swelling and speeds up healing.

There are several homeopathic remedies such as mercurius solubilis or belladonna that may be used if the glands are infected and sore. Baryta carbonica may be recommended if they are merely enlarged but otherwise not causing you a problem. Other remedies include a clay poultice to draw out the fluid, and aromatherapy oils such as chamomile, thyme, mint, and lavender.

AIDS (Acquired Immune Deficiency Syndrome)

Knowledge about AIDS is expanding so rapidly that any "facts" or figures given today may not be valid a year or even a few months from now. But, with that in mind, we will attempt to give at least an overview of the disease as it is known today, and an idea of what you might do to protect yourself from contracting it.

As of early 1987, about 30,000 people in the United States have been diagnosed with AIDS, and another 1.5 million are thought to be carriers. Eighty-five nations have reported cases of AIDS, and the World Health Organization estimates that between 5 and 10 million people worldwide are infected with the virus. They also estimate that in the next ten years up to 100 million people could become infected.

The disease, which was once thought to affect only male homosexuals, drug users, and a few unfortunate transfusion recipients, is now showing up in the heterosexual population too.

The test which identifies the AIDS carrier is the HTLV III antibody test. It is a blood test which is available through most large clinical laboratories. The main problem with the test is that the blood levels of the AIDS antibody don't become high enough to give a positive reading until four to six months after infection. So one negative test within six months of contact doesn't necessarily mean that you're safe. During the period between infection and the production of sufficient antibodies to show up on the test, you are, however, infectious.

Worse still, new data indicate that at least 50 percent of the people testing positive on the antibody test go on to develop full-blown AIDS. As greater numbers are diagnosed and followed up, doctors are finding that a larger and larger percentage are eventually developing the disease.

AIDS is of course so far incurable by conventional or alternative methods. It is so lethal because it attacks the immune system, paving the way for "opportunistic" infections such as a type of meningitis, pneumonia, and a type of skin cancer called Kaposi's sarcoma. It can lodge in the brain, resulting in nervous system degeneration. If you are pregnant you can pass it on to your unborn baby.

First symptoms are night sweats, fever, extreme weight loss, lethargy, and a general feeling of being unwell, followed by swollen lymph glands and skin blotches.

However, with all the panic news articles it is important to put AIDS into perspective. First, it's only passed through the blood or intimate sexual contact. You can't catch it by being in the same room as an AIDS carrier, or by shaking hands with a hemophiliac. Second, those who do succumb to the illness are usually below par—that is, their immune systems are in poor shape to begin with. As we've seen elsewhere in the book, this can have a lot to do with your life-style and other factors. The risk is higher if you or your partner sleep around, if your male partner is or has been bisexual, or if you or your partner is a drug user or hemophiliac.

Conventional AIDS treatment consists of the use of powerful antiviral drugs, chemotherapy, and Interferon, an anticancer drug.

The most publicized of the new antiviral drugs used to fight AIDS is azidothymidine (AZT). In most patients it was given to during testing, the drug prolonged survival and caused clinical improvement such as increased energy, weight gain, and improved mental function in the patients to whom it was given. AZT, however, is not a cure and is very toxic. It causes bone-marrow damage and severe anemia in some patients. Also, to be effective, it needs to be taken every four hours, around the clock.

♫ How can you avoid contracting AIDS, and what does alternative medicine have to offer?

Prevention includes the avoidance of casual sex. Get to know your partner before leaping into bed with him and don't be afraid to check him out for sexually transmitted diseases—this is where your assertive techniques come in! It's also worth following "safe sex" guidelines such as using a condom and spermicides, and avoiding anal sex. Don't share a razor or hypodermic syringe with anyone else.

Alternative approaches to AIDS focus, as you would expect, on building up the immune system. Previous viruses or bacterial infections, which have involved the use of a lot of antibiotics, may have impaired your immune resistance. Leon Chaitow, in an article in *Here's Health* (March 1986), suggests that there is a connection between *Candida albicans* (yeast) and AIDS:

"The frequent use of antibiotics leads to candida proliferation and damage to the normal flora of the bowel (and) also to changes in the control of substances passing from the bowel to the bloodstream. Bowel permeability is altered and this allows undesirable proteins to enter the system, leading to allergies as well as to a drain on immune function."

Diet, as you would expect then, is the mainstay of any alternative approach. A naturopathic regimen of diet and supplements is suggested to rid the body of *Candida*, and boost the body's defenses.

Stress reduction techniques, acupuncture to rebalance the body's self-regulating system, and herbal medicine are also said to be helpful.

Graham Hancock and Enver Carim, the authors of *AIDS: The Deadly Epidemic* (Gollancz, England) describe significant remissions in two sufferers who undertook a holistic program of diet, exercise, positive thinking, acupuncture, and visualization techniques. AIDS patients at St. Mary's Hospital, London, are using visualization techniques to try and stimulate healing of their damaged T-cells. In an article in *Homoeopathy Today* (1985/6) a medically qualifed homeopath outlines the possibility of treating AIDS with remedies such as tuberculin, homeopathic vaccines such as carinii for pneumonia, and preparations (nosodes) made from the patient's own cancerous tissue or body fluids.

It's only fair to say that neither alternative nor conventional therapies have cracked the AIDS problem, but natural therapies can provide a useful adjunct or even a complete alternative to the more usual treatments.

For further information, contact:

The AIDS Action Council
Phone: (202) 547-3101

This is a lobbying organization but should have information on groups in your area.

Pelvic Inflammatory Disease

Pelvic inflammatory disease (PID) is an umbrella term for a number of pelvic infections. It can be the result of sexually transmitted diseases such as gonorrhea or chlamydia, or other vaginal infections, birth complications, a septic abortion, or a complication of IUD use. It can cause painful periods. And it's estimated that in 20 percent of infertile couples the reason for failure to conceive is scarring of the fallopian tubes due to PID.

Symptoms are low abdominal pain, increased menstrual pain, discharge, a high temperature, pain on intercourse, irregular bleeding, and general flulike symptoms. As the results are potentially so serious, you shouldn't try to treat yourself. Get help as soon as possible. Generally, antibiotics are the best primary treatment. They are mandatory if the infection is due to gonorrhea or chlamydia.

Alternative therapy in this instance is ancillary, aimed at supporting the immune system, improving general health, and relieving stress and pain. A whole food diet, herbal medicines, homeopathy, and visualization may all be helpful. Chiropractic and osteopathic manipulation, and acupuncture, will help relieve congestion and pain in the pelvic area. Many naturopaths use herbal drawing packs to help establish drainage from the infected area. Hot sitz baths will also help drainage and are good for pain relief.

PID can become chronic if inital therapy was inadequate or begun too late. Some women with chronic PID have constant pain, and others have a periodic recurrence of their symptoms, usually when they're run down.

Orthodox treatment of chronic PID is generally less effective than it is for acute PID. Prolonged use of antibiotics, of course, increases the possibility of yeast infection and can have other unpleasant side effects. Surgery to remove the infected tissue is the last resort. Unfortunately, "the infected tissue" is often the uterus, fallopian tubes, and ovaries. Alternative therapies are similar to those recommended for acute PID.

A whole food diet with abstinence from coffee, tea, sweets, and alcohol is advised. Increasing vitamins C, A, E, and zinc is helpful but should be done under the guidance of a nutritionally oriented practitioner or naturopath. Herbals such as echinacea, golden seal, and thuja help fight infection and build up the immune system. The herbal drawing pack is often useful in chronic PID if the site of infection has not become walled off by adhesions. Visualization and stress reduction techniques can help reduce frequency and severity of recurrences.

Osteopathic and chiropractic manipulation may improve blood flow and nerve conduction in the area, and thus increase the effectiveness of other treatments. Acupuncture will often help relieve pain and balance energy flow, as can reflexology and shiatsu.

Keep in mind that both acute and chronic PID are serious diseases, and that while combinations of the above therapies have worked well for some cases, other women may need antibiotic and even surgical intervention.

For further information:

Check with your local women's health clinic, Planned Parenthood, or your doctor to see if any local support groups exist.

Cystitis

Eight out of ten of us suffer this miserable condition at some time in our lives. Fortunately for most of us it's an isolated event. But for an unlucky few it keeps coming back, and life becomes an endless round of antibiotics, which more often than not result in yeast infections and the need for further medication.

Symptoms are wanting to empty your bladder frequently but producing little urine, burning or stinging when you pass urine, low abdominal pain, or backache, and sometimes bloodstained urine.

In some cases, cystitis is caused by infection. But for about 50 percent of women, urine analysis shows no sign of bacteria. Triggers are wide-ranging— they can include sex, alcohol, tea and coffee, too much sugar in the diet, heat and cold, wearing tight clothing, prolapse, chemicals in soap, bubble baths, the swimming pool, or spermicides—and that's just a few. Some of us experience minor cystitis just before a period.

♂ Orthodox treatment

This consists of antibiotics, and sometimes a preparation called potassium citrate (Pot. Cit.) to rebalance the pH level of the urine, plus advice to drink plenty of fluids and to rest. Very occasionally women may be given a "urethral stretch" which seems to alleviate symptoms for some.

But about one in ten women who experience repeated attacks resist antibiotic treatment, and for them the medics have coined the term "urethral syndrome." So what has alternative medicine to offer? And is there anything you can do to help yourself?

♂ Self help and alternative treatment

As in many other conditions, stress makes cystitis worse. There are a number of things you can do to help prevent cystitis, and alternative therapies can also be very effective in treating it. Herbs such as uva ursi, buchu, and chimaphila, and the homeopathic remedies apis mellifica and cantharis can both be helpful in overcoming cystitis. Diet is important: citrus fruits, sugar, alcohol, coffee, and black tea can aggravate bladder and urethral symptoms.

Recently, it has been found that allergy plays a role in some recurrent cystitis. For these people, certain allergens will cause all the symptoms of full-blown cystitis, but no bacterial cause is found in the urine culture. Allergy testing and avoidance of offending substances or desensitization by injection or sub-lingual drops can be very effective.

Aromatherapy, consisting of compresses and massage as well as warm baths, can be helpful: cedarwood and pine may be especially useful.

Osteopathy or chiropractic may be able to iron out certain anatomical pro-blems that may predispose you to cystitis. For instance, some lower back condi-tions may cause bladder irritation.

Acupuncture also works very well in cases of cystitis. Biochemic tissue salts can be a first line in an emergency: Ferr. Phos., Kali. Mur., Kali. Phos., and Mag. Phos. are the suggested remedies, depending on your symptoms.

To prevent an attack

☞ Eat a good whole food diet.

☞ Drink three to four pints of liquid a day, but stay away from tea and coffee. Herb teas and mineral waters are better.

☞ Don't wait if you want to empty your bladder; go to the toilet regularly.

☞ Don't use vaginal deodorants, bub-ble baths, talc, and perfumed soap.

☞ Pay attention to hygiene. Wash after moving your bowels, using plain cool water.

☞ Wipe your bottom from front to back to prevent germs from the anus entering your urinary tract.

☞ You and your partner should wash before sex.

☞ Empty your bladder before and as soon after sex as you can. Wash your genital area too by pouring cool water over it so as to flush out any germs that may have entered while you were making love.

☞ Avoid love-making positions that put pressure on the bladder. Positions where you are on top, or your partner enters from behind may be better than the good old missionary.

☞ Don't make love until you are well aroused, so as to avoid vaginal dryness. If for any reason your natural secretions are scanty (for example, after menopause) use aloe vera gel for lubrication.

☞ Practice pelvic floor exercises to generally strengthen the area.

☞ Avoid tight pants and wear cotton underwear. Watch what you wash your underwear in—no highly scented detergents.

☞ Some find that keeping the urine acidic helps prevent cystitis attacks. This can be accomplished by drinking a glass of cranberry juice each day and avoiding citrus fruits and tomatoes.

If you develop an attack

🍂 At the very first twinge, increase your fluid intake. Drink half a pint of water every 20 minutes for three hours.

🍂 Drink barley water to soothe inflammation.

🍂 Stay warm. Place a hot water bottle wrapped in a towel against your back or pelvic area, or take a hot bath.

🍂 The most common bacteria causing cystitis, *Escherichia coli,* tends to make your urine alkaline and does best in that environment. Cranberry juice in large quantities, about a quart a day, helps turn the urine acid and discourages its growth.

🍂 Avoid citrus fruits, tomatoes, and melons. They are very alkalizing and will increase your discomfort.

🍂 Steer clear of coffee, tea, alcohol, sweets, and anything spicy.

🍂 Take lots of vitamin C. The excess is excreted in your urine and helps fight the infection.

🍂 Use a tea of equal parts uva ursi, buchu, and marshmallow root—at least four to six cups a day. Herbal tinctures can be very useful, but these are best prescribed by an herbalist or a naturopath.

🍂 If you do have to have antibiotics, make sure you get plenty of vitamin C, since they rob your body of this vitamin. Eat plenty of yogurt to rebalance your system, or take acidophilus tablets.

Benign Breast Disease

Cancer has such a high profile that it's hardly surprising that many of us panic when the slightest thing goes wrong with our breasts. Do bear in mind that 75 percent of breast lumps are absolutely harmless. Especially if you are under forty most breast problems are due to what doctors call "benign breast disease."

🍂 Lumps and bumps

Many of us experience tender, lumpy breasts just before a period, especially during our teens and in the years preceding menopause. The lumpiness, which seems to be a result of the way the body reacts to its own hormones, passes once your period is over and is nothing to worry about.

As you get older, more definite lumps or cysts may appear. Fibrocystic disease is the rather vague term sometimes used to describe these. Occasionally, the doctor will drain the cyst to make sure it isn't malignant—more often than not it's safe to leave it alone. A lump that is harder to diagnose is a fibroadenoma.

Though a combination of mammography and ultrasound can often give a doctor a pretty good idea of whether or not a lump is cancerous, the only way to be sure in the case of a solid lump is to remove and biopsy it.

Other less common signs of benign breast disease are nipple discharge, nipple retraction, and skin problems like eczema. Nipple discharge, although alarming, is not usually serious. It may be white, creamy, green, yellow, clear, or even bloodstained. It's usually the result of a noncancerous lump in the ducts (ductal papilloma). Surgery will usually be advised to rule out the possibility that the lump is cancerous.

The usual orthodox approach to benign breast disease is hormones, analgesics, and as already described in some cases, surgery.

⨍ What has alternative medicine got to offer?

A broad-based dietary approach can help enormously. There's quite a lot of evidence that benign breast disease may be a result of allergy. Excess caffeine seems to play a part, so cut out coffee, tea, and cola-type drinks if you are prone.

Evening primrose oil, already described under PMS, will reduce swelling and pain for many women. Homeopathy and herbalism can help correct hormonal imbalances.

On a practical level, wear a good supporting bra, and get plenty of exercise to stimulate circulation to the breasts. Yoga may be especially helpful—try the bow and cobra postures. For others, consult your yoga teacher.

Homeopathic dosages of estrogen and progesterone have been given to some women, with what one practitioner describes as "a number of useful outcomes." The treatment isn't widely available as yet, but if you are interested consult a clinical ecologist.

The symptoms of benign breast disease and cancer can be the same, so if you do develop a breast problem, don't delay seeing your doctor or a medically qualified alternative practitioner. But, as we said at the outset, the vast majority of these problems aren't usually serious. Don't be afraid to ask your practitioner exactly what is wrong—for your own peace of mind.

Cancer

ℐ Can you prevent cancer?

Cancer prevention involves following three simple rules:

ℐ As far as possible, avoid exposure to cancer-causing substances such as tobacco, chemicals at work, additives, and so on.

ℐ Adopt a healthy life-style—the tips for staying healthy in Part One are useful here. A diet rich in vitamin A is said to be especially useful.

ℐ See your doctor if you develop any of the following:

☐ a sore that doesn't heal

☐ an unusual lump or thickening

☐ unusual bleeding or discharge

☐ a change in a wart or mole, for example, itchiness, bleeding

☐ difficulty in swallowing or persistent indigestion

☐ persistent hoarseness or a cough

☐ a change in your usual bowel habits

ℐ Breast cancer

Breast cancer. The very words make many of us quail. It's hardly surprising. One in eleven women develops breast cancer. And the disease is still the number one killer of women aged forty to fifty. Despite new forms of treatment, the five-year survival rate for breast cancer remains at 50 percent, regardless of treatment. What's more, this figure has barely shifted in the last fifty years. This is because in 50 percent of all women operated on for breast cancer, the cancer has spread to other parts of the body.

But all is not complete doom and gloom. Orthodox medicine now claims a 90 percent twenty-year cure rate for very early breast cancer. The catch is that these are cancers which are only a few millimeters in size. Anything large enough to be felt in a clinical exam has most likely spread to the lymph nodes. This re-emphasizes the importance of using mammography and ultrasound imaging, as already outlined, as a routine screening method for women over forty.

Because breast cancer is so common, it's well worth thinking about it *now*; then if you should ever need to, you will be in better position to make the choices that are right for you.

So who gets breast cancer? Is there anything you can do to reduce your chances of developing it? And if you are diagnosed as having breast cancer, what sort of help is available?

Risk factors for breast cancer

You stand a higher chance of getting breast cancer if you fall into one of the following groups:

- ☐ You have no children.
- ☐ You have your first child over the age of twenty-five (some experts say thirty).
- ☐ You began your periods early.
- ☐ You have a late menopause.

- ☐ Your mother, grandmother, sister, or other close female relative has had breast cancer.
- ☐ You are overweight.
- ☐ You have a history of cancer in the other breast or elsewhere in the body.

You'll see the factors that put you at an increased risk of developing breast cancer in the list above. That's not to say that if you fall into this high-risk group you are bound to get the disease. But if you are in this category, it will certainly pay to be extra careful and well informed, in order to avoid unnecessary additional risks, and so that you can seek early treatment if you do get breast cancer.

How can I tell?

The incidence of breast cancer increases with age. The commonest symptom is a lump or deformity in the breast. Look out for any dimpling or a retracted nipple that isn't normal for you—especially if the nipple is pulled in all around, rather than just in a strip across the nipple. Contrary to conventional wisdom, pain *can* be a symptom of breast cancer, especially if you are past menopause. Nipple discharge is also a sign, and very occasionally there are no symptoms at all. That's not to say that any of these symptoms *is* breast cancer. As the section on benign breast disease showed, all these symptoms can also indicate far less serious problems. Even so, you'd be wise to consult your doctor or a medically qualified alternative practitioner if you do experience any of them.

The commonest place to find a lump is the upper, outer quadrant of your breast, followed by the upper, inner quadrant, or the underside of the breast.

See your doctor if you develop any of the following:

☐ Change in the shape or size of one of your breasts.

☐ Puckering or dimpling of the skin.

☐ Enlarged veins.

☐ Lump or thickening of breast tissue.

☐ Nipple discharge.

☐ Retracted nipple.

☐ Change in skin texture or rash on the nipple.

☐ Swelling of the upper arm or armpit, or above your breast.

☐ Noncyclical breast pain.

Diagnosis

The doctor will examine your breasts and may be able to hazard a fair guess if the cause of the problem is breast cancer. You will then be sent for mammography (a special breast X ray). If cancer is suspected, a biopsy, which involves taking a sample of the diseased tissue, will confirm the diagnosis. This may be done by aspiration (when a small sample is sucked out through a fine needle), or by removing the lump. Further investigations to ascertain the type of cancer and how far it may have spread can include blood tests, X rays, and sometimes an estimation of liver function.

It is frightening to be told you have breast cancer. Do bear in mind that breast cancer is not just a disease that women die from. Many of us live with it for many years. And though neither alternative nor orthodox therapies can claim to have conquered breast cancer, it is something that can often be controlled. The most important thing is that women who want to do so can keep some control over what is happening to them. The more you know about treatment options, the more you can cooperate and decide on the sort of treatment that will suit you best.

Orthodox treatment

At one time anyone diagnosed as having breast cancer would automatically expect to have her breast removed. However, studies have shown that mastectomy or more extensive breast surgery, as opposed to just removing the lump, does *not* necessarily lead to longer survival, (though the risk of the cancer recurring in the affected breast is higher if the lump alone is removed). This risk can be reduced by follow-up treatment with radiation therapy.

Your options will depend on the type of cancer and whether there is any evidence that it has spread elsewhere in your body.

In early breast cancer, where the lump is a few millimeters in diameter and there is no evidence that it has spread (metastasised), surgery is the primary treatment. This can take several forms:

⫘ Lumpectomy—where the lump and a small area of surrounding tissue are removed.

⫘ Partial mastectomy—where a larger part of the breast is removed.

⫘ Total mastectomy—where the whole of your breast and the lymph glands are removed but the underlying muscles are left.

⫘ Radical mastectomy—where the whole of the breast, the lymph glands under the arm, and the underlying muscles are removed. This is much less often performed today than in the past.

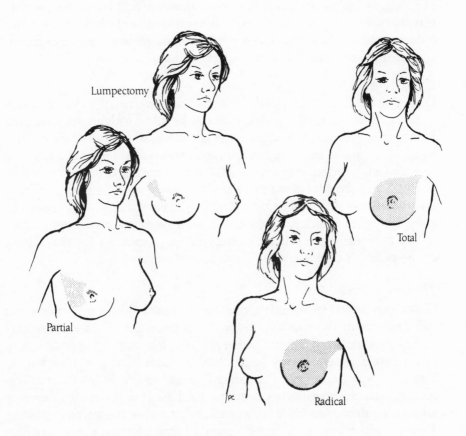

Types of masectomy.

Where there are several lumps or a large part of the breast is affected, mastectomy may be the best surgical treatment, or you may prefer it to prevent the chance of cancer occurring again in the same breast, or if you want to avoid radiation therapy.

Back-up treatment (adjuvant therapy)

This is aimed at wiping out any remaining cancer cells.

Radiation therapy
A carefully controlled dose of radiation is aimed at the cancer site. The snag is that the X rays can't discriminate between cancer cells and noncancer cells, and the treatment has several unpleasant side effects such as exhaustion, nausea, and skin soreness that usually appear after two to three weeks. What's more, the body can only take so much radiation, which has the effect of lowering the body's immune defenses. Sometimes radioactive metal wire implants are used to provide booster doses of radiation to the bed of the lump.

Chemotherapy
Drugs that kill the cells as they divide (cytotoxic) are given, the idea being that as cancer cells divide very rapidly they can be killed without destroying the healthy cells. The biggest drawback is the side effects, which include nausea, hair loss, loss of appetite and taste, weakness, numbness of the fingers and toes, and anxiety. Combinations of cytotoxic drugs reduce the risk of death over a five-year period by about 9 percent for certain groups of women. However, the treatment is less useful for women over fifty and the costs and benefits need to be carefully weighed in each particular case. New "targeted" cytotoxic drugs designed to bind only onto cancer cells themselves offer the promise of a way around some of the problems of side effects. These are not yet available.

Hormone treatment
Tumors that depend on estrogen to grow can be treated with an antiestrogen drug called tamoxifen. This is usually the first line of treatment if you are over seventy or have problems such as heart disease, which might make an operation risky. Alternatively, tamoxifen may be given for a couple of years as a back-up to surgery or other treatment. The reduced rates of relapse in women over fifty seem to make this a worthwhile treatment for those of us in this age group. Side effects seem to be relatively few; they include hot flashes, nausea, and vomiting. However, it's only fair to say that no one yet knows what the long-term effects of such treatment may be.

Treating the ovaries

As we've already said, many breast cancers are estrogen-dependent. It would seem to follow that preventing the ovaries, which produce most of the body's estrogen, from working might have the effect of reducing the tumor. This is occasionally done either by removing the ovaries (oophorectomy), or by destroying their action by radiation. This seems to help in women past menopause. If you are younger than this, such a procedure will cause early menopause, and an increased likelihood of heart disease, since the female hormones protect women against heart problems.

Decision time

You may be the sort of person who is happy to hand yourself over to your doctor and let him or her decide on treatment. On the other hand, several studies suggest that counseling and understanding can do much to reduce anxiety and distress. Try to find out as much you can about your cancer, what stage it is at, and how far it may have spread, as well as your specialist's favored treatment methods. Discuss possible side effects. It can be hard to think straight, and remember what questions you want to ask when you are feeling worried, so take along a friend or partner and make a list of questions.

Remember, many lumps have been there for several years before discovery. A couple of weeks' delay while you explore the pros and cons of different forms of treatment isn't likely to make much difference in the success of your treatment.

Where cancer has spread

If your cancer has spread, treatment will be aimed at controlling symptoms, preventing it from recurring elsewhere, and keeping you in as good health as possible. Treatment again will depend on your age, where the cancer is, and the length of time between inital treatment and spread. Hormone treatments alone may be offered; chemotherapy, hormone injections, and radiation therapy can all be part of the treatment.

Life after mastectomy

For most of us our breasts are very important. In a world where our mammaries are used to sell everything from newspapers to cars, it's hardly surprising that we should see them as symbols of our sexuality. We feed our babies with them and we get sexual pleasure from them, so the loss or disfigurement of a breast may lead to deep feelings of loss. Complete removal of the breast, as we said earlier, is much less common today. If you do have this done it's important not to bottle up your feelings. Talk them over with a nurse, doctor, skilled counselor, or friend. Give yourself time to grieve and expect to feel angry, depressed, and confused. It's all part of the mourning process.

Breast reconstruction

The words "breast reconstruction" can make your body sound a bit like a building site. An implant can be put in at the time of the original operation or later, or you may be offered a prosthesis. Where the cancer is small and doesn't appear to have spread, this can be very successful, and may help you regain a sense of identity. However, some women feel that the rush to recreate what was there is a way of avoiding coming to terms with the illness, and seeing its meaning. They argue that in a world where women are often judged purely on appearance and sexual attractiveness, treating breast cancer as merely a cosmetic problem that can be corrected as simply as a face-lift is a way of denying the importance of the experience. That's not to say that it might not be right for some of us, but do give the matter some careful thought before jumping at the chance of prosthesis.

Future checkups

You'll be given regular checkups to make sure all is still well after the initial treatment. It's natural to feel worried, and to find all sorts of lumps and bumps before going for a checkup. Taking along a friend, and being open about your feelings, will help.

♫ Genital cancers

Cancer can occur in the vulva and vagina, cervix (neck of the womb), the body of the uterus, the ovaries, and the fallopian tubes. Of these, cervical cancer is by far the most common, and cancer of the fallopian tubes the least. Cancer of the uterus usually occurs between the ages of fifty and sixty, and you are at greater risk of developing it if you have diabetes or are overweight. Cancer of the ovaries also occurs mainly in older women. Cancer of the vulva and vagina is relatively rare.

Cervical cancer

Cancer of the cervix is commonest between the ages of forty-five and fifty, but recently the age at which it occurs has been creeping down. Normal cervical cells undergo certain precancerous changes, and if the condition can be nipped in the bud, treatment is virtually 100 percent successful. If it progresses, treatment is much more difficult. Because of this, the traditional focus has been on detecting these changes early by means of a Pap test, otherwise known as a cervical smear.

Pap test

A Pap test is a simple, painless test in which a few cells are taken from the neck of your womb and are analyzed for precancerous changes.

In screened populations, there has been a 50 percent or greater decrease in invasive cervical cancers. In view of these statistics, it is clear that the small inconvenience and cost of getting regular Pap tests is well worthwhile.

How often should I have a Pap test?

Expert opinion is divided. It used to be thought that every five years should be the recommended time between tests. Today experts are more likely to suggest that most women be tested every year, while those in a high-risk group should have a smear every six months.

What if I have a positive test?

It can be frightening to be told your test is positive. Remember—it doesn't always mean you have cancer. It usually means that some of the cells have changed in such a way that they could lead to cancer if they continued to undergo such changes. We don't know how often cells do change and return to normal. But it's a fact that often the cells will revert to their usual state. Regular Pap testing may be all that is required.

More severe changes in the cells will be treated. You'll be given a colposcopy (examination of the cervix with a microscope) to see the extent of the changes. The cells will then be destroyed by using a laser, freezing them off, or carrying out a cone biopsy, in which a small part of the cervix is removed under anesthetic. After a cone biopsy you'll experience some bleeding. Your cervix may be weaker after the operation, and if you go on to become pregnant you may need a special stitch to avoid miscarriage.

Incidentally, if you have an abnormal test you don't have to give up sex. It can't make the condition worse, and you can't pass it on to your partner. Making love can be a valuable source of comfort when you are feeling worried.

Pap smears are graded from I to V. Class I is normal; any class above this is increasingly abnormal, with V being carcinoma. Class II smears are often simple inflammatory changes due to infection or some trauma to the cervix.

These often revert to normal on their own but do need to be watched. Of course, it's a good idea to treat any infections which may be causing the inflammation. Class III and IV smears are more serious. Here the cells have become somewhat abnormal. These abnormal or dysplastic cells are not cancerous, but there is evidence that they may represent a transitional phase between normal and cancerous cells. While mildly dysplastic cells may return to normal, more severely affected cells do best with treatment. Orthodox treatment consists of destroying the abnormal cells with cryosurgery, laser surgery, or cone biopsy. These are generally effective in eradicating the dysplastic cells, but they can lead to cervical scarring.

In the rare event that cancer has progressed farther than this, treatment is by surgery, radiation therapy, and in more advanced cases, chemotherapy.

Am I at risk?

Women who are at the greatest risk of developing cervical cancer are:

☐ Those who have had several sex partners, or whose partner has had several sex partners.

☐ Those who smoke, or occasionally, whose partners smoke.

☐ Those who have genital warts (HPV) or whose partner has genital warts.

☐ Those with a large family, especially if you started your family early.

☐ Those with husbands who work in "dirty" or dusty jobs such as miners, metal workers, leather workers, or those who work on machines or with certain chemcials or textiles.

Preventive tips

✍ Barrier methods of contraception such as the condom, diaphragm, or cervical cap are thought to offer some protection against abnormal cervical changes. (One study showed that in women with positive tests whose partners started using a condom the cells went back to normal.)

✍ Immunity can be lower as a result of stress or lack of vitamins. Concentrate on stress reduction techniques, yoga, meditation, relaxation, and exercise. And make sure you have a good diet.

✍ You and your partner should keep your sexual organs clean. It's a good idea for the man to wash before sex.

✍ If you or your partner develop genital warts, herpes, or chlamydia, make sure you get treatment, and make a point of having regular Pap smears.

See your doctor if:

☐ You develop any abnormal bleeding from the vagina.

☐ You experience an unusual or offensive vaginal discharge.

☐ You suffer unexplained weight loss or a swollen abdomen.

☐ You develop an ulcer on your genitals that fails to heal, or any unusual lump or bump.

Orthodox treatment for genital cancers consists of surgery, plus chemotherapy and/or radiation therapy as a backup.

The alternative approach to dysplasia

As you may expect, the alternative approach to treating dysplastic changes is aimed at improving general health and reducing stress. General diet and vitamin therapy are used, as are stress reduction techniques and visualization.

Two specific treatments for mild to moderate dysplasia are large doses of folic acid (a B vitamin), and an herbal drawing pack applied weekly to the cervix. Folic acid has been shown to help dysplastic cells revert to normal. And the herbal drawing pack helps slowly kill the dysplastic cells and stimulate healing. Both of these therapies should be carried out by a naturopath or nutritionally oriented doctor. It's a good idea to have Pap tests every three months during treatment to keep track of how you are doing. If you see no progress in six months or if the dysplasia gets worse, you should probably go with the orthodox treatment.

♊ The alternative approach to cancer

It's clear that orthodox medicine doesn't have all the answers where cancer is concerned. While conventional treatment is undoubtedly effective in treating some forms of cancer such as blood, skin, lymph gland, testes, and cervix, if carried out early enough, in other cases treatment is distinctly hit or miss. Breast cancer, other than very early lesions, is an obvious example, where as already observed, survival rates have remained at 50 percent despite advances in treatment and detection. Surgery removes the lump, and chemotherapy may kill cancer cells, but they damage the immune system and, as we've seen, may have unpleasant side effects.

An increasing body of evidence suggests that all of us have cancer cells in our bodies at times during our lives. In most cases our immune systems swing into action to fight off the disease before it has a chance to take hold. For some reason, in people who develop cancer, this fails to happen. The observation that those who have undergone severely stressful experiences, such as bereavement or divorce, have lowered immune resistance, and are therefore more likely to fall prey to cancer, offers some valuable clues as to why some people should be at risk. Resistance may also be lowered by diet, genetics, and hormonal or environmental factors.

Most alternative practitioners take the view that cancer is not merely a disease of the cells, but a disease of the whole person. This approach is summed up by the director of the charity New Approaches to Cancer who told me "Our approach to cancer is that cancer is a deeper problem within a person and unless the deeper problem is resolved then the cancer will more than likely appear in another area if only treated by conventional methods." The alternative approach, as you'd expect, is geared to the whole person rather than to treatment of any particular form of cancer. What's more, it doesn't distinguish between male and female cancers, although as the director of New Approaches to Cancer says again: "One aspect of our approach that we would see very applicable, particularly to breast cancer, would be that of emotional trauma, either acute through loss or separation, or chronic through non-existent or disturbed relationships."

Because alternative approaches to cancer set out from a different starting point than does conventional medicine, it's very difficult to compare one treatment with the other. Holistic G.P. Dr. Patrick Pietroni, in an article in the medical journal *Cancer Topics* (Sept/Oct 1986) wrote: "It would be fair to say there there is no objective evidence as yet that any of these techniques add to longevity for any one group of patients. However, *nearly all studies remark on the improvement in quality-of-life and the relationships surrounding the patient, his (sic) family and advisors.*"

So, if you want to undertake alternative treatment for cancer, it would be wise not to go into it with the view that it will *cure* you. What it can do is to help you to sort out the meaning of your cancer for you personally, and perhaps alleviate symptoms.

Incidentally, a study is now taking place at the Bristol Cancer Help Centre in England to compare five-year survival rates of women with breast cancer who have undergone orthodox and alternative treatment, so we may soon have some more definite answers to the question: "Does alternative medicine help in cancer?"

The immune system link

Once again, the immune system and its relation to the rest of our body is the cornerstone of the alternative approach. An increasing body of clinical evidence lends weight to the suggestion that stress lowers the body's immune resistance and so encourages cancer growth.

The main aim of all alternative treatments is to boost your body's defenses. Cancer being the end result of a long degenerative process, you shouldn't try to go it completely alone. Find a sympathetic practitioner and let your doctor know.

What can I expect?

The main emphases, from an alternative position, are diet and the influence of mind and spirit on the body. Homeopathy, herbal medicine, and acupuncture also all have something to offer.

Is there a cancer personality?

Several studies now show a connection between cancer and personality. Holistic practitioner Laurence LeShan lists the following characteristics that he has found to be common to cancer patients:

- Unsettled childhood.
- Low opinion of yourself.
- Unsatisfactory relationship with your parents.
- No creative outlets.
- Keeping a tight lid on your emotions.
- A defeatist attitude.
- Loss of an important relationship.

It could be said that in our society almost anyone will have experienced one or more of these. And many people would argue that such a classification leads to victim-blaming and guilt. Nevertheless, loss does have a crucial part to play in depression, as you'll see in the mind-body chapter. Women especially experience loss in a particular way, because so often they see themselves in relation to others around them, rather than as autonomous beings.

According to the studies just mentioned, cancer patients are of a particular personality type. Basically they are "nice" people. The argument goes that when such a person experiences a major loss, the body's immune system becomes depressed and fails to cope with cancer cells. A study at King's College Hospital, London, showed that the five-year survival rate among women with breast cancer depended critically upon attitude. Patients with a fighting spirit, or those who denied that they had cancer and just got on with life, survived more than twice as long as those who simply gave in. A large dose of optimism, or refusal to give in, apparently stimulates the body's antibody system.

It's only fair to say that such research is still in its infancy, and, not surprisingly, many orthodox oncologists (cancer specialists) dismiss it completely. One leading cancer specialist, writing in the doctor's magazine *Pulse*, states "Cancer of the breast has an unpredictable course; at one extreme patients may die within a month of diagnosis and at the other, patients with advanced disease may live for many years. By carefully selecting the type of case, evidence can be accumulated that any treatment can prolong life." However, the same specialist is forced to concede that much orthodox medicine retains practices that are completely unscientific as well as potentially dangerous and invasive.

Visualization

A visualization technique, pioneered by Carl and Stephanie Simonton, incorporates breathing, relaxation, meditation, hypnosis, and positive thinking. The idea is that you are encouraged to think of the cancer cells as "weak and confused" and to focus on the stronger healthy cells in your body fighting them off. To give you an idea of what this involves, we quote a passage from the book *Love, Medicine and Miracles* (Harper & Row) by Dr. Bernie S. Siegel: "I told my body to be well. I told my immunological system to protect me. I looked at my brain, my bones, my liver and my lungs every night. I felt them and told them to be free of cancer. I watched my blood flowing strongly. I told the wound to heal quickly and the area around it to be clean. I told my other breast to behave, because it's the only one my husband and I have left. I still tell my body and mind every night, 'I reject cancer. I reject cancer.'"

Such visualization techniques are enormously flexible. You can use any images that suit you. You don't have to use the language of attack. In fact, as Dr. Siegel points out, the "war model" of cancer may in fact be inappropriate since the cancer cells are your own cells gone astray. Imagining your white cells engulfing the cancer cells, or eating them, may well be more appealing images.

The meaning of cancer

An important part of the alternative approach to cancer is to help people discover the meaning that cancer has for them. Illness, and cancer is no exception, can make it easier to say no to things we don't want to do, or to escape from the demands placed on us by others. This may be especially significant for women who both have to conform to the often contradictory and unrealistic expectations placed on them by society, and find it difficult to say no. Illness can be a way of getting the love or nurturance that we may feel unable to ask for in any other way. It's reasoned that once you know what psychological needs the illness is serving, you can begin to satisfy them in different ways. Ann Oakley, whom I quoted earlier, vividly recreates the meaning that cancer of the mouth had for her in her book *Taking it Like a Woman* (Flamingo): "To have a cancer in my mouth was a direct attack on my identity. Given the importance of words in my work I needed my mouth, not primarily to speak, but to think in words, to write. It was where I lived. It was the source of my vitality, my creativity . . . and also a site of my sexuality. Because of this, one of the first things Robin did when the diagnosis of cancer was made was to kiss me."

At the Bristol Cancer Help Centre in England, and other places using alternative approaches to cancer, a lot of emphasis is placed on cancer as a "transformational experience" that can change your whole way of experiencing life. Ann Oakley says again: "It became clear to me that living in the present does have to do with knowing who one is, but that it also has to do with appreciating that timelessness denied by the modern world in its preoccupation with superficial change and senescence, with making a friend of eternity."

Finally, although reports of "cures" are purely anecdotal, as Patrick Pietroni points out in the article mentioned earlier: "Those few anecdotal reports on spontaneous regression in cancer all describe what has been termed 'a dramatic existential shift' . . . involving a resurgence of hope, together with an alteration in belief system and acceptance of responsibility for the process of healing and recovery."

The diet connection

If you've read this far you won't be surprised to discover that the other mainstay of the alternative approach to cancer is diet. A report by two orthodox oncologists in 1981 attributed one-third of all cancers to diet. Many alternative practitioners would put the figure much higher.

The key, certainly where women's cancers are concerned, may lie in some connection between hormones and diet. Breast cancer is far more common in countries where fat intake is high, for example. What's more, as discussed earlier, estrogen plays an important role in female cancers of all kinds. Breast cancer rates are higher in women who began their periods early and who had a late menopause, and who therefore have high levels of circulating estrogen for longer. It's known too that estrogen is stored in body fat. A recent study published in the journal *Cancer* reports that women with breast cancer have higher levels of estradiol (a form of estrogen) in their bloodstreams than the control group they were compared with. What's more, a report which appeared in the *American Journal of Clinical Nutrition* in 1984 points to the significance of diet in length of menstrual cycle. White women fed on a meatless diet had fewer periods. The report suggests we should look at the possibilities of using vegetarian diets in post-menopausal cancer patients.

Women with positive Pap smears have been discovered to have diets containing less than 30 mg of vitamin C a day. This could help explain why women who smoke seem to be at higher risk of developing cervical cancer, as smoking robs the body of vitamin C (as does the Pill). Low levels of vitamin C have also been associated with breast cancer.

Other studies have linked low levels of vitamin A and beta carotene, a type of vitamin A, to the development of cancer. The Hunza tribe of northern Pakistan, who eat a diet high in B_{17} (found in dried apricots, the kernels of cherries, apricots, apple pits, and so on), are remarkably free of cancer, though, so far as we know, no one has studied the social factors in this community, which may help explain their apparent resistance to the disease. A study in the *British Journal of Cancer* has shown that women with early cancer of the cervix had less beta carotene in their bloodstreams than did a control group. Vitamin E and the mineral selenium have also been implicated in the prevention of cancer.

As always, the story is far from clear-cut, and we don't yet known how these nutrients may serve to protect against cancer, or how useful they are in treating it. Vitamin A, for example, may block the effect of carcinogens in the breast and reproductive system, and may also prevent the body from converting cancer-causing chemicals into toxins.

As you would expect, fiber too seems to play a large part in preventing cancer. Many studies have shown that those with cancer consumed less fiber and more sugar than healthy control groups. This can perhaps be explained by the fact that fiber binds cancer-causing substances in the body and speeds their progress through the gut.

One other point that is perhaps less often mentioned in dietary studies is what effect our manner of eating our food has on us. Patrick Peitroni in the article quoted earlier describes a study carried out in Ohio on rabbits, which found a 60 percent reduction in the formation of arterial problems in a group of rabbits fed a high fat diet: "This group of rabbits were being fed by a different laboratory technician who insisted on taking each rabbit out of its cage, calming and stroking it before it was fed a high fat diet."

Is it too fantastic to reason that humans too might benefit from a calmer state of mind at mealtimes? Might this explain why some people, in spite of an apparently poor diet, don't go on to develop cancer or heart disease?

Diets for the treatment of cancer

Dietary treatments for cancer include a whole range of approaches—fasting, detoxification, the use of supplements, injections of laetrile (an enzyme found in apricot kernels which is thought to explain why the Hunzas are resistant to cancer), and coffee enemas.

Two of the most famous dietary regimens are the Gerson diet and the Bristol diet, developed at the Bristol Cancer Help Centre. Briefly, the Gerson diet works on the principle that cancer patients have a low immune response and generalized tissue damage, especially of the liver. When cancer is eliminated by whatever method of treatment, poisonous wastes appear in the bloodstream. These eventually destroy the body unless they are disposed of. The diet aims to regenerate the body and to stimulate its self-healing mechanisms. It's an extremely rigorous regimen, which includes no tap water, smoking, or alcohol, and women aren't allowed to use make-up. However, a five-year study, carried out in Australia, of patients where cancer had spread to the liver shows several unexpected partial remissions.

The Bristol Cancer Help Centre Diet adheres to the following principles:

☞ No meat.

☞ Mainly raw food.

☞ No junk food.

☞ No coffee or tea. Two glasses of wine or a measure of spirits are allowed each day, as they are thought to stimulate the production of beneficial prostaglandins.

☞ No salt.

☞ The inclusion of sprouted seeds rich in B_{17}. (There's been some recent controversy about this since sprouted alfalfa has been found to contain substances that suppress the immune system. Adherents of the Gerson regimen have now abandoned sprouted seeds altogether, but the Bristol Centre rejects this advice.)

☞ Vitamin supplements of A, B, C, and E. (But not vitamin E for hormone-dependent breast cancers.)

☞ Mineral supplements of magnesium, potassium, calcium, zinc, and selenium.

As always then, the message seems to be to cut down on fat, sugar, and processed foods and to step up your intake of fresh foods, fiber, vitamins, and minerals.

For further information:

Of course, it's impossible in a book this size to do full justice to the complexities of the various dietary methods. I suggest you read *You Can Conquer Cancer*, by Ian Gawler (Thorsons).

Other alternative cancer treatments

These include the use of iscador (mistletoe) in homeopathic doses or herbal preparations. Other herbal treatments for cancer include those that work on the liver, such as burdock, blue flag, yellow dock; on the lymphatic system, such as cleavers, echinacea, and poke root, and other herbs such as sweet violet.

TENS (transcutaneous electrical nerve stimulation) and acupuncture can play a part in pain relief, and spiritual healing is an important art of treatment in alternative cancer centers.

You may want to undertake alternative treatment in conjunction with orthodox medicine, either as a preliminary to surgery and the rest, or as a backup. Only orthodox practitioners can prescribe specific cancer treatments, of course, and it's here that we come up against the difference of approach between orthodox and alternative therapists again. Most alternative practitioners would claim not to be treating the cancer, but the whole person.

Alternative cancer treatment review

☑ Diet.

☑ Relaxation.

☑ Yoga, T'ai Chi.

☑ Megavitamin therapy.

☑ Counseling and/or psychotherapy.

☑ Exercise

☑ Avoidance of chemicals in the environment, e.g., aerosol sprays.

☑ Creative expression, e.g., art therapy, dance therapy.

☑ Acupuncture or TENS.

☑ Spiritual healing.

☑ Meditation/visualization techniques.

Before deciding on treatment, become familiar with the type of orthodox treatment available, and its success rate in treating your particular type of cancer.

It doesn't hurt to get two or three opinions here. If the orthodox treatment is usually successful, it's probably best to go with it and use alternative therapies as a backup. If, however, the rate of cure is poor and the treatment entails a lot of discomfort and expense, you may want to rely more heavily on alternative therapies as a way of at least improving the quality of your life, if not the length of your survival.

Before we end this chapter—a word of warning. Do remember that if you have cancer your body has broken down in a big way and has more than likely been weakened further by aggressive surgery or drugs. Any alternative treatment you undergo is going to take time—and no one can expect miracles. Inevitably, many people with cancer aren't cured, any more than they would be by orthodox methods. However, a large number who have undergone alternative therapy testify to the improved "quality" of their lives. Perhaps we should end this chapter with two quotations that we hope sum up the spirit of what we have written. The first comes from a cancer patient writing in the British magazine *Spare Rib*; the second is from American feminist Audre Lorde, whose *The Cancer Journals* (Sheba) is well worth reading: "If we keep fit and survive long after the medicos think we can—what does it matter which treatment worked? "I would never have chosen this path, but I am very glad to be who I am, here."

For further information, contact:

> The International Association of Cancer Victors and Friends, Inc.
> 7740 Manchester, Suite 110
> Playa del Rey, CA 90293

> National Women's Health Network
> 224-7th St. SE
> Washington, DC 20003
> Phone: (202) 543-9222

Mental Health
☔ The size of the problem

Doctors' offices are crammed with people who are visiting not because of any physical condition but because of emotional disturbance. Of course, such disturbances can affect people physically, as was shown in the section on stress. Sometime during their lifetime, most people will find themselves with a mental health problem and will see a doctor. Of these, women are twice as likely to complain of depression. If you are a married woman you are more likely to suffer from anxiety than a married man. And two-thirds of agoraphobics are women. Why?

Anxiety and depression are often the end products of stress overload, and as we saw in Part One, there are many aspects of women's lives that predispose them to stress. Women are encouraged to express their feelings more openly than are men. Whereas a man who is feeling depressed or anxious may be inclined to take refuge in excessive drinking or sex, or keep a stiff upper lip, women are more likely to make their way to the doctor's office. What's more, in our jobs as mothers and wives, we are more likely to have direct contact with the medical services, so this may seem the obvious place to seek help for emotional problems.

Depression is often initiated by a loss of some kind—perhaps the loss of a job, a partner, or a cherished belief. That's not to say that everyone who experiences any sort of loss automatically becomes depressed. And, of course, a period of depression and mourning can be a perfectly natural and appropriate response to certain aspects of life, for instance, following a marriage breakup. But there are some factors that make women more vulnerable. Loss of another person is likely to be experienced as a terrifying loss of part of a woman's self or purpose in the world. And the loss of a job may threaten the already tenuous hold a woman feels she has on the outside world, increasing her doubts about her rights and abilities to function outside the domestic sphere.

According to this view, depression isn't so much an illness as a result of things going wrong in our lives or relationships.

A psychologist who has carried out research into some of the reasons for depression writes in the journal New Scientist: "The reason that more women than men, and more people of lower socio-economic status . . . become depressed is quite simply that women and working-class people on average have lives with more possibility of things going seriously wrong, and fewer social and economic possibilities for dealing with the kinds of things that do go wrong."

It's difficult to draw a distinct line between anxiety and depression, since they tend to be two sides of the same coin. You may experience more symptoms connected with one than the other, but both may well be present. Psychologists have sometimes argued that depression is more concerned with our feelings about the past, while anxiety has to do with fears for the future.

∬ Are you at risk of depression?

Research shows that those who are most at risk of getting seriously depressed include:

☐ those with no paid work outside the home;

☐ those with preschool children;

☐ those with three or more children under fourteen living at home;

☐ those with a low income;

☐ those without the support of an intimate relationship;

☐ those who have suffered a loss or bereavement early in life (especially loss of the mother before the age of eleven).

∬ What sparks depression?

Depression can be triggered by many things, including:

∬ Genetic factors.

∬ Life events (for a list of these see the Holmes-Rahe scale in the section on stress).

∬ Psychological factors. Some psychologists attribute depression to "learned helplessness," when we feel so out of control of our lives and it seems pointless to even try. Others attribute depression to "faulty thinking," i.e., the way we view the world affects our moods. Psychoanalytical theories see depression as a result of aggression being turned inward upon ourselves.

∬ Biochemical imbalances. For instance, an essential amino acid, tryptophan, has been found to be low in those suffering from depression.

∬ Environmental pollution and allergies.

∬ Low blood sugar.

∬ Drugs, including "social" ones like alcohol.

∬ Illnesses such as a bout of flu, mononucleosis, etc.

∬ Accident or injury.

∬ Surgery, e.g., mastectomy.

∬ Fatigue and overwork.

∬ Menstrual problems.

∬ Loss of a job through retirement or layoff.

∬ Divorce and separation and the ensuing loneliness.

⨌ When to seek help

The point at which a depressed or anxious mood, which all of us suffer from time to time, becomes "illness" is a moot one, but if you've been experiencing any of the following for longer than a couple of weeks, consider going to see your doctor or an alternative practitioner:

☐ You have no appetite and may have lost weight.

☐ You feel constantly tired and all your get-up-and-go got up and went.

☐ You can't get to sleep at night or you wake up early in the morning.

☐ You feel agitated and on edge much of the time.

☐ You can't summon any interest in things you used to enjoy.

☐ You feel guilty and blame yourself for things that go wrong.

☐ You have difficulty concentrating and are more indecisive than usual.

☐ You've had thoughts of ending it all.

⨌ Orthodox treatment

When it comes to mental disorders there are signs that the conventional medical world is beginning to take social explanations more seriously. A recent article in the medical journal *The Practitioner* states: "Patients with minor depression, vulnerable personalities or immediate life stresses can be helped by careful analysis of the problem, discussion and counseling." Nevertheless, treatment with antidepressants and tranquilizers is still the first line for more long-standing episodes of depression, the idea being that these can correct biochemical disturbances that are present in the brain in depression.

Antidepressant drugs come in two types—the tricyclics which are used for moderate to severe depression, and the mono-amine oxidase inhibitors (MAOIs), which are prescribed if the tricyclics haven't worked. The main problem with these drugs is that they don't *cure* depression. They work by acting on biochemical changes in your brain that are present in depression, with the result that your sensitivity to emotions is reduced. What's more, they don't work for one out of three people.

And they take up to four weeks before they start to take effect. In the meantime, there may be several unpleasant side effects, including drowsiness, dry mouth, visual difficulties, nausea, constipation, shaking, rashes, sweating, and sex and bladder problems, to mention a few. The MAOIs react with certain foods containing tyramine, such as cheese, broad beans, meat, or yeast extracts, and certain red wines and sherry. That's not to say that these drugs can't be helpful for getting us through a difficult situation. But in the long run, masking the symptoms of depression can't cure broken nights, a crying baby, insufficient money to live on, or an unsatisfactory relationship with your partner. By encouraging you to define your problems as an "illness," these drugs can prevent you from trying to change things for the better or coming to terms with them.

If your doctor does prescribe a drug, make sure you know exactly what it is, why it's being prescribed, what side effects you can expect, how long you will have to take it, and how to come off it. Some of the effects of coming off antidepressants can be extremely severe and frightening, especially if you are not expecting them and if you have been on the drugs for a long time.

Tranquilizers

𝕀 One in five women takes tranquilizers or sleeping pills at some time in the course of each year.

𝕀 Middle-aged women and those over seventy-five are most likely to be on tranquilizers.

𝕀 Tranquilizer use is higher for women who don't work outside the home.

Tranquilizers are frequently prescribed for anxiety, and for difficulty sleeping at night. The trouble is, tranquilizers are often prescribed for problems directly related to poor housing, lack of money, loneliness, and so on. As one expert on tranquilizer use has put it: "When the G.P. prescribes tranquilizers he's putting *you* out of *his* misery."

Tranquilizers can certainly be effective in the short term. But research shows that as time goes on they lose their efficiency. Even more seriously, if you've been on tranquilizers for a long time and then try to come off them suddenly, you may experience a whole range of unpleasant and frightening withdrawal symptoms. And, as with antidepressants they can keep you from tackling the real problems that lie behind the symptoms of anxiety.

There simply isn't space in a book of this sort to go into detail on the question of tranquilizers. Seek further information from books, friends, a nutritionist, or a local women's health group. Always be prepared to *ask your doctor* the following questions, should he or she prescribe tranquilizers (or any other medication) for you:

1. WHAT AND HOW?

☞ What kind of tablets are they?

☞ How can they help me?

☞ How should they be taken?

☞ How can I see if they work?

2. HOW IMPORTANT?

☞ How important is it that I take them?

☞ What may happen if I do not take them?

3. WHAT SIDE EFFECTS?

☞ Do they ever cause trouble?

☞ Do they have any side effects?

☞ Can I drive after taking them?

☞ Can I take other medicines with them?

☞ Can I drink alcohol when I am taking them?

4. HOW LONG?

☞ How long must I continue with these tablets?

☞ What should I do with tablets I do not need?

☞ Will I need to see you again?

☞ What will you want to know when I see you again?

Coming off tranquilizers

☞ Take it slowly. It's better to cut down gradually than to try to do it all at once.

☞ See a nutritional therapist or ask your doctor to recommend a vitamin and mineral supplement.

☞ Pay attention to your diet.

☞ Find out if there is a local support group in your area (contact your G.P. or local health education department).

☞ Give yourself time.

☞ Be realistic. Don't expect it to be easy and don't punish yourself if you slip up from time to time.

☞ Relaxation, massage, and visualization can all help.

☞ Get other people on your side so that they know how you are feeling and are aware of any difficulties you are having.

☞ Acupuncture may help you give up your addiction—but only if you really want to in the first place.

☞ If you feel the urge to take a pill, distract yourself—phone a friend, go for a walk, do some exercise, practice yoga or meditation.

☞ Try herbal treatment.

This is just the barest outline of a complex subject.

For further information:

Bottling It Up, Valeri Curran and Susan Golombok (Faber and Faber).

Coming off Tranquilizers: A Withdrawal Plan That Really Works, Shirley Trickett (Thorsons).

Nutrition and Mental Illness, Dr. Carl Pfeiffer (Thorsons).

✎ Alternative approaches to mental health

Given the side effects and other problems of orthodox treatments for mental problems, what does alternative medicine have to offer?

This area is one in which almost any of the alternative therapies can prove useful, even some that on the surface may seem unpromising, such as acupuncture. A woman acupuncturist quoted in *Dealing with Depression* by Kathy Nairne and Gerrilyn Smith (Women's Press) says: "The needles by themselves can do much to calm agitated energy or to raise it in cases of physical or mental depletion. There are specific treatments which in some cases can reestablish balance almost miraculously in people who are seriously disturbed . . . However in many cases a rearrangement of lifestyle is necessary if the treatment is to be effective."

The final sentence is perhaps an explanation of why the alternative therapies can be so helpful. Following the guidelines laid out in Part One of the book can provide a useful basis.

As always, *diet* plays a large part in the alternative approach. Professor Bryce-Smith of Reading, England, has written on the role zinc deficiency may play in depression. The amino acid tryptophan has been found to be low in people suffering from depression. Taking supplements of this seems to result in improvements that can be usefully compared to standard antidepressant drugs. This is one "alternative" therapy you may be able to get from an orthodox doctor. You shouldn't take it if you are on MAOI antidepressants, as it can cause eyesight problems and headaches, nor should you take it if you are suffering from bladder disease.

Homeopathy has a large number of remedies, which as always, are linked to particular personality types.

On the *herbal* side, infusions such as lemon balm, oats, vervain, or chamomile are helpful in mild cases. More powerful herbal remedies can be very useful; you should consult a qualified herbalist or naturopath for suitable remedies.

Most of the *mind-body* therapies such as yoga, meditation, the Alexander technique, and relaxation programs can help, as can various types of psychotherapeutic techniques outlined in the last part of the book.

For further information on the role of alternative therapies in treating mental disorders, contact:

The Huxley Institute
900 North Federal Highway
Suite #330
Boca Raton, FL 33432
(305) 393-6167

PART THREE

Fertility and Reproduction

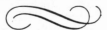

Contraception

Like it or not, most women's lives are bound up with their fertility. The whole question of reproduction is one that has been medicalized to the nth degree. Better family planning methods have been responsible for women's greater longevity—very few of us die in childbirth nowadays—for smaller families, and for the fact that women today can be more independent than their grandmothers. On the face of it there is more choice than ever before in contraception. Yet some of us—and it is overwhelmingly women who take the responsibility for contraceptive measures—find it difficult to choose what is the best sort for us.

All present contraceptive methods have their drawbacks, and the type of contraception you need will depend to a large extent on your age and the stage of your life. For instance, if you don't have sex very often, it's pretty pointless to be on the Pill. If you just want contraception to space children, rather than because you have finished your family, your priorities in choosing a method will be different. The whole issue is even more complicated because the Pill, which at one time seemed about to herald a new age of freedom, has come under ever-growing suspicion on health grounds. This section looks at orthodox contraceptive methods, and then looks at the viability of natural family planning methods as an alternative.

♫ Orthodox contraceptive methods

Barrier methods, e.g. diaphragm, cervical cap, condom

Effectiveness
Varies between 85 and 99 percent depending on how carefully you use them.

Safety

Extremely safe, although some women are allergic to rubber or spermicides. Condoms offer some protection against sexually transmitted diseases and cervical cancer. Cystitis is sometimes a problem with some types of diaphragms.

Advantages

Flexible, especially if you aren't engaging in sex very frequently. Can be used long or short term. Helps you to get used to handling your own body and to feel at ease with it.

Disadvantages

May interfere with spontaneity. Some couples dislike using a spermicide and find it messy and unaesthetic. Some men complain that a condom reduces sensation during lovemaking. May be implicated in vaginal infections.

The Pill

Effectiveness

Very effective. The combined Pill is 99 to 99.9 percent effective. The mini-Pill (progestin only) is 96 to 98 percent effective.

Safety

An increasing body of evidence points to quite considerable disadvantages. The most recent studies suggest a connection between the long term use of the Pill and breast cancer. However, the Pill seems to offer some protection against ovarian cancer, and cancer of the body of the uterus.

Think very carefully about taking a high-dose Pill if any of the following apply:

☐ You have a history of thrombosis.

☐ You have had cancer of the breast or reproductive organs.

☐ You smoke.

☐ You get migraines.

☐ You have existing high blood pressure.

☐ You are diabetic.

☐ You are overweight.

☐ You have severe varicose veins.

☐ You are over thirty-five.

☐ There's a family history of thrombosis or hyperlipidemia.

Advantages

Extremely effective if you definitely don't want to become pregnant. Its action is continuous so you can have sex any time without the fear of getting pregnant. It doesn't interrupt lovemaking.

Disadvantages

Reduced effectiveness if you have had a bout of diarrhea, forget to take it, or are on certain drugs, e.g., antibiotics. Side effects range from those which are a nuisance—such as weight gain, depression, loss of sexual desire—to high blood pressure, migraines, gall-bladder disease. Cancer risk as already outlined. Associated with higher rate of cervical erosion. Depletes the body of several important nutrients, e.g., vitamin C, zinc. Sometimes makes PMS worse.

Intrauterine contraceptive device (IUCD or IUD)

Effectiveness

About 97 percent if you have already had children, slightly less if you haven't.

Advantages

Once it is in place you can forget about it, only needing to replace it every one to five years, depending on type.

Disadvantages

Can make your periods heavier and more painful. Increased risk of pelvic inflammatory disease (PID) which can impair future fertility. PID is apt to occur with IUD use if you are younger and have more than one sexual partner. If you get pregnant while using an IUD, there is an increased risk of ectopic pregnancy or miscarriage. In rare instances an IUD may perforate the uterus. It may be expelled without your noticing.

Progestins

Depo-Provera or Noristerat. A form of progestin is given as a long-lasting injection which lasts for two to three months.

Effectiveness

Extremely effective—over 99 percent.

Advantages

Once it's been done you can forget about it.

Disadvantages

Can't be stopped if you change your mind. Drug stays in your body eight to ten months. Can cause either heavy, irregular bleeding or stop periods altogether. Side effects include weight gain, headache, depression, backache, reduced sexual desire, nausea, abdominal discomfort, acne. May take up to two years before fertility returns.

Collatex sponge

Effectiveness

From 75 to 91 percent as far as is known.

Advantages

May be more comfortable and less messy than diaphragm. Because it contains spermicide, repeated intercourse can occur without the need for extra spermicide. No fitting required—one size fits all.

Disadvantages

As for other barrier methods. But, unlike diaphragm, sponge should not be used during a period. May cause vaginal dryness and irritation.

Morning-after Pill (post-coital contraception).

A special high dose Pill is used within three days of unprotected intercourse (two tablets followed by another two, twelve hours later).

Effectiveness

Said to be 99 percent effective.

Safety

If the method fails, hormones could affect baby.

Advantages

Avoids having to have an abortion.

Disadvantages

Side effects are severe, and may include nausea and vomiting, and withdrawal bleeding. Should not be used routinely, but only when you suspect your practised method of birth control may have failed.

Sterilization

Either vasectomy for men or tubal ligation (when fallopian tubes are clipped, tied, or cut) for women.

Effectiveness

Virtually 100 percent.

Disadvantages

Some women experience heavier, more painful periods or irregular bleeding. You can't count on reversing the process, although microsurgery can reverse some vasectomies and ligations.

For further information:
Check with Planned Parenthood in your community.

⌁ Alternative methods of family planning

The risks and drawbacks of conventional family planning methods already outlined have led many to explore natural family planning methods. It's important to distinguish between the new natural techniques and the old-fashioned "rhythm" method, which well earned the tag "Vatican roulette" because of its high failure rate.

The new techniques are neither haphazard nor unscientific—they are based on careful and accurate observation of the signs and symptoms of fertility. However, they do demand a degree of dedication and self-discipline that some women find irksome.

How does it work?

Natural family planning techniques make use of the fact that you are only fertile for about three days each month. In fact, over your whole lifetime you are fertile for a mere 4 percent of the time. Given the relatively restricted time during which conception can occur, natural family planning experts argue that taking precautions every single time you make love is like using a sledgehammer to crack a nut.

Natural family planning methods based on careful observation of the fertile period are in theory, *and when used properly*, as effective as the Pill in preventing an unwanted pregnancy. The biggest bonus of course is that they are entirely free of side effects.

Fertility awareness

The key to natural family planning is fertility awareness. That means having a basic knowledge of the way in which your body prepares itself for pregnancy each month, plus an understanding of your partner's potential fertility.

Once the ovum is released it has a lifespan of twelve to twenty-four hours. If it is not fertilized by the sperm during this time, it dies and is reabsorbed by the body. Your partner, on the other hand, can be 100 percent fertile from puberty onwards. The life of a sperm can be anything from a few hours to up to five days, during which it can fertilize the egg if conditions are favorable.

Whether a sperm survives and makes it to the egg depends on the mucus produced by your cervix under the influence of estrogen and progesterone. Immediately after your period, estrogen levels are low and the discharge produced by the cervix is very scanty and thick. As ovulation gets nearer, estrogen levels rise, and the cervix produces a mucus which is clear, slippery, and favorable to sperm: it both nourishes the sperm and creates "tracks" along which they can move rapidly toward the uterus. Estrogen levels peak about forty hours before the egg is released and then fall.

A few days after ovulation, estrogen begins to rise again but progesterone production predominates. The mucus again becomes hostile to sperm and conception cannot occur. The potential fertility of you and your partner therefore depends on the lifespan of the egg combined with the lifespan of the sperm. Natural family planning means you can work with the natural cycle, either abstaining from sex or using a barrier method during the short period when conception can occur.

There are two main methods of natural birth control: the mucus method and the sympto-thermal method.

The mucus method

This is also known as the ovulation or Billings method and relies on the observation of mucus changes already outlined. It is basically a method of determining impending ovulation before it happens. The first day of a period is counted as day one, and since it is virtually impossible to detect mucus during menstruation, this is considered a potentially fertile time. After a period most women experience a "dry" spell when there is no mucus or the the mucus produced is scanty, thick, opaque, and hostile to sperm. The fertile phase begins when wet mucus appears, especially wet, thin, stringy mucus. You can detect the mucus either by wiping your vaginal entrance with a tissue before going to the toilet, or by inserting a finger and taking a sample from the cervix.

As ovulation approaches, the mucus becomes increasingly favorable to sperm. It is wet and lubricative and can be stretched between thumb and forefinger like raw egg white. Ovulation usually occurs within two days of the appearance of this type of mucus. After that it becomes thick, sticky, and clotty or disappears altogether.

According to this method, you are potentially fertile during your period and during the "wet" days, plus an extra four days to allow for the lifespans of the sperm and egg and the possibility of a second ovulation (when this occurs it's always within 24 hours of the first). The last days of the cycle, about ten days in all, are infertile. The phase of the cycle leading up to ovulation can vary a lot from woman to woman and from month to month, and it is this variation which is responsible for the different lengths of cycle we all experience. The second phase of the cycle—from ovulation to menstruation—is almost always fourteen days.

Observation of mucus can be especially useful if you are breast-feeding and have not yet restarted your periods, as it can tell you whether you are ovulating, which is useful if you don't want to get pregnant again soon. Fertility usually returns gradually as the baby has fewer breast feedings and this may be marked by "patchy" mucus, indicating that the body is trying to ovulate.

The sympto-thermal method

The sympto-thermal method combines mucus observations with recordings of temperature changes. The addition of temperature readings enables one to determine the safe time *after* ovulation. In addition, you are encouraged to notice other cyclical changes such as breast tenderness, alteration in the position of the cervix, mood changes, and so on. Using all this information it is possible to pin down the fertile period with a fair amount of accuracy.

The basis of the sympto-thermal method is temperature recording. The lining of the uterus has been compared to an incubator which every month gets warm and ready to receive a baby, under the influence of progesterone. The resting temperature of the body (basal body temperature, or BBT) is recorded at the same time every day. During the early part of the cycle, under the influence of estrogen, the BBT remains low. After ovulation the presence of progesterone in the bloodstream causes a rise in BBT. If you don't become pregnant, your temperature will drop again either just before or during your period. If you do conceive, the high level of circulating progesterone which continues for the first three months of pregnancy causes your body to maintain a higher temperature. For this reason, changes in temperature can be used as an indicator of pregnancy long before either chemical tests or physical examination would show up as positive.

The rise in temperature is only slight (about 0.4 to 0.6°F) so it is a good idea to use a specially calibrated basal body thermometer (available from large drug stores) rather than the ordinary fever kind, which is more difficult to read and not detailed enough.

A good time to take your temperature is first thing in the morning *before* getting up. You can take it by mouth, vaginally, or rectally. Since an ovum lives for twelve to twenty-four hours, you should avoid unprotected intercourse for two whole days of higher temperature. In other words you need to have recorded *three* higher temperatures.. Women who use the method say taking daily temperature readings becomes such a habit that it is no more bother than cleaning your teeth or brushing your hair.

In addition to temperature and mucus observations you may notice other signs of ovulation. Many women experience pain or a small amount of mid-cycle bleeding when they ovulate. Another good indicator is the position of the cervix. During the early part of the cycle the cervix is low and you can touch it with your finger. The opening, or *os*, is closed and the cervix is firm. Toward ovulation the cervix is pulled higher into the vagina by the ligaments which support it. The os opens slightly, especially if you have had children, and the cervix softens. Other signs of the later part of the cycle include such premenstrual symptoms as bloating, weight gain, breast tenderness, and emotional changes.

For your interest, there are two other methods of fertility control that are dependent upon cycles rather than implements. *Lunaception* is a method of contraception that determines ovulation by the moon. *Astrological birth control* is based on the idea that your fertile period is determined by the angles of the sun and moon in the sky at the time of your birth.

If you are curious enough to look into either of these approaches to natural family planning, they are best coupled with some sort of rhythm method, as there is no firm evidence in support of their efficacy.

Special circumstances

Childbirth

If you've just had a baby it can be difficult to observe fertility signs, especially if you are up several times a night, and generally overtired. As soon as the lochia (the discharge after the childbirth) has stopped, you can start observing mucus again. If you are breast-feeding completely on demand and frequently, you are unlikely to be fertile, but keep up your observations so that returning fertility doesn't catch you unaware.

Vaginal infection

A vaginal infection will make observation of mucus difficult, especially if you are using any creams, suppositories, or ointments to treat it. You can continue to take your temperature and start checking mucus again as soon as you are sure the infection has completely healed.

Premenstrual syndrome

Because of hormone imbalances that may occur as part of PMS, your mucus patterns may be somewhat irregular. Treating your PMS according to the guidelines laid down earlier may make fertility signs easier to identify. Since PMS symptoms are often made worse by the Pill and the IUD, natural family planning methods may be especially suitable if you are a PMS sufferer.

Further advice on dealing with special circumstances is available in the books listed at the end of this section. Of course, the big question is "Does it work?" Dr. Anna Flynn, a leading expert on natural family planning, says, "As with all types of contraception the success or failure of the methods depends on how much the couple want to avoid pregnancy." In theory, the effectiveness of the sympto-thermal method is 99 percent, but most sources rate the user effectiveness of the method at 89-94 percent. These figures compare favorably with more established methods such as the diaphragm, condom, and the sponge. The secret of success seems to be strong motivation and good teaching. A short chapter such as this can't do more than lay down the basic outlines of the method. For furter detail either get one of the books mentioned, or better still attend a natural family planning course.

There are only two physical circumstances in which natural family planning techniques might be impracticable. The first is if you have a cervical erosion, since this produces a discharge which may mask the cervical mucus. The second occurs when the cervix has been cauterized, since this can alter mucus production.

There are various kits and gadgets on the market that can aid fertility awareness. However, they are all a bit expensive, and despite new advances many are somewhat hit or miss. Most natural family planning experts would argue that though such gadgets may be useful, they are no real substitute for knowing your own body's individual patterns.

For further information:

Fertility Awareness Workbook, Barbara Kass-Annese & Dr. Hal Danzer (Putnam Publishing Group).

Natural Birth Control, Katia and Jonathan Drake (Thorsons).

Contraception Naturally, Francis J. Trapani (CJ Frompovich).

To find a teacher in your area, contact:

Los Angeles Regional Family Planning Council
3250 Wilshire Boulevard, Suite 320
Los Angeles, CA 90010

Center for Health Training
2229 Lombard St.
San Francisco, CA 94123
or your local Women's Health Center.

Infertility

About one in six couples has difficulty conceiving. In fact the term "infertile" is perhaps inaccurate, since in many cases the problem turns out to be "subfertility." In other words, they are able to conceive but for one reason or another, for instance, sexual difficulties, stress, or malnutrition, the system needs a bit of a kick to get it into action.

Infertility problems have increased in recent years—the reasons for this increase include the fact that more of us are putting off having a family until over age thirty, when fertility is starting to decline, and that the incidence of sexually transmitted disease has increased (outlined earlier in the book).

The whole field is an area in which orthodox and alternative views and practices cross each other. Many orthodox practitioners would agree that modern drugs and environmental chemicals play a part in reducing fertility, either because they affect the absorption of nutrients from the diet, which are necessary for a healthy hormone balance (for instance, too much cadmium may result in a zinc deficiency, which has been linked to male infertility), or because they affect the sperm or egg directly.

✍ What are the main causes of infertility?

For women:

✍ *Damaged fallopian tubes, ovaries, or uterus*. This usually results from a previous infection inside or outside the tubes, following a ruptured appendix or pelvic abscess, from complications following a miscarriage, abortion, or difficult birth, or from endometriosis. More rarely, the tubes have been malformed from birth. Signs that your tubes may be damaged are pain during intercourse, general pelvic aching, and irregular or heavy, painful periods.

✍ *Endometriosis* (see vaginal infections for further details). This is when tissue that normally lines the womb implants in other parts of the body. The main symptoms are pain during intercourse and heavy and painful bleeding.

✍ *Hormone imbalances* resulting in failure to ovulate or irregular ovulation. Possible symptoms are short, irregular, or absent periods.

✍ *Problems affecting the cervix and uterus*. Cervical infection or erosion can cause subfertility. Some cervical mucus is "hostile" to sperm, preventing it from passing into the uterus. Fibroids can also affect the ability to conceive or carry to term.

✍ *Being very overweight or underweight*, which affects the hormone balance.

For men:

✍ *Low sperm count or no sperm*. This may have been caused by orchitis secondary to mumps; the effects of certain drugs; surgical damage—for instance, from a hernia operation—the sperm being stored at too high a temperature because of an undescended testicle; overweight; wearing tight jeans and pants; sexually transmitted diseases; or a hormonal imbalance. Just as women are sometimes allergic to their partner's sperm, men too sometimes form antibodies against their own sperm; finally, making love too often can lower the sperm count.

✍ *Poor quality sperm*. This can result from hormonal imbalance; varicocele—a sort of varicose vein of the testes; or hydrocele—a bag of fluid in the scrotum; inflammation of the prostate gland; or too much or too little semen.

✍ *Blocked tubes* caused by scarring from infection or sexually transmitted disease, or where the tubes are twisted.

Other factors

These include various medical conditions such as TB or other severe illnesses; disorders of the endocrine system, like diabetes; infections of the genital or urinary systems such as yeast or cystitis. Then there are sexual problems of a physical or emotional origin—for instance, in the man, the failure to achieve or maintain an erection, in the woman, a vagina that is too tight or goes into spasm during intercourse. Even something as simple as sexual technique can be to blame for some problems. The sperm needs to be deposited high in the vagina if it is to stand the best chance of entering the cervix and fertilizing an egg. Sexual positions where the penis can penetrate deeply are best. For conception to occur, ideally the semen should bathe the cervix for at least half an hour after intercourse, so obviously if you leap up and wash yourself immediately after making love you aren't really giving nature a fair chance. This may present you with a problem if, for example, you suffer from cystitis, which is why it's worth getting such problems cleared up before trying to conceive.

What treatment is available?

A full medical history and examination will be carried out on both of you. The whole business may be rather depressing, and you could well be letting yourself in for a whole series of tests and investigations spanning several years.

Semen analysis or sperm count

This is the first and most basic test carried out on the man. It involves your partner masturbating into a clean container. The sperm will be tested for their mobility and shape, to make sure they are normal. Usually this is done several times over a period of months.

Post-coital test

Cervical mucus is examined after intercourse to see how easy it is for sperm to move through, i.e., to determine whether it is hostile or too thick.

Further male tests

These include measurements of gonadotrophin levels and tests to see whether your partner is infertile for genetic reasons.

Ovulation tests

These include several of the techniques already outlined in natural family planning, i.e.,
1. taking your temperature daily
2. cervival mucus test
3. measurement of hormone levels

Endometrial biopsy

A scraping of tissue is taken from the lining of your uterus to see if ovulation has taken place.

Laparoscopy

This surgical procedure enables the doctor to look at your ovaries, fallopian tubes, and uterus. The abdomen is inflated with carbon dioxide so that space exists between your pelvic organs. Then an instrument like a periscope (laparoscope) is passed through a small cut near your navel. This enables the surgeon to check for fibroids, endometriosis, and blocked fallopian tubes.

Hysterosalpingogram

This test shows the position of any obstruction in the tubes, and the internal structure of the uterus, by means of a water-soluble dye which is injected into the cervix. A series of X-ray pictures which will show the site of any blockage is then taken.

♫ Orthodox treatment

The sort of treatment you will need depends on your medical history and the results of the various tests. Sometimes all that is necessary is to clear up local infection, or get simple advice on timing of intercourse. Simple self-help techniques like douching the vagina to make it more alkaline (for example with bicarbonates such as baking soda) or acid (see vaginal infections) can make the environment more favorable to sperm. Men can be helped by simple advice to wear loose fitting underwear and avoid tight jeans or trousers; bathe the testes in cold water every day; cut down on alcohol; or go on a diet. Often, simple measures such as these do the trick.

Where these don't work there are two main lines of treatment—hormonal and surgical. Both of these have progressed by leaps and bounds during the last few years. The commonest "fertility drug" is Clomid, which is taken daily from the second to fifth days of your cycle to stimulate ovulation. Pergonal is a combination of gonadotrophins (hormones released by the pituitary) which is given by injection. It's the drug that tends to stimulate multiple pregnancy if not given in a very carefully controlled dose. Newer techniques involve "hormone releasing factors" which control ovulation, administered by means of a small portable pump, about the size of a cigarette pack, that is strapped to your arm or leg.

Hormone treatment for men is less successful, though some men have been successfully treated by using human chorionic gonadotrophins of the sort used to stimluate ovulation in women. And there is hope that hormone releasing factors may be of use to men too.

Surgery involves operations to remove fibroids or cysts if they are interfering with conception, or to correct any abnormalities of the reproductive system. Some of the most dramatic advances recently are in the area of tubal micro-surgery, which seems to offer a better chance of unblocking tubes, reshaping the entrance to the tube, and removing scar tissue (adhesions) than more conventional techniques.

Other methods of treating infertility include test tube fertilization (IVF) in which embryos fertilized outside the woman's body are placed in the uterus by means of a fine tube and artifical insemination (either by husband or by an anonymous donor—AIH and AID, respectively).

Alternative approaches

Despite the successes of modern medicine in treating infertility, a small number of couples find themselves unable to conceive, often for no apparent reason. This can be where alternative techniques come in.

Stress reduction

Stress seems to play a major part in many cases of unexplained infertility— hence the common experience of couples who conceive immediately after they have started adoption proceedings. A *relaxation and exercise program* as outlined in Part One of the book can certainly help. *Hypnosis* has recently been shown to be effective in some women experiencing repeated miscarriage. The stress that undergoing treatment can have on a relationship shouldn't be ignored either. One couple makes the following point in an article in *Mother and Baby* magazine, October 1984: "Infertility is an enormous strain on a relationship. At first it's easy to laugh at having to have intercourse to order, but that palls after a while and you begin to feel a freak. Talking to other people and realiz-ing there are others in the same boat eases the pain." *Joining a support group* such as Resolve Inc. can help. *Meditation* and *yoga* can be useful too.

Diet

Eating a good whole food diet, cutting out coffe and tea, and not smoking can help. One study in the *BMJ*, June 8th, 1985, showed that even as few as ten cigarettes a day can reduce fertility.

Supplements

Some experts advise supplementation with *vitamin* C and amino acids such as arginine for low sperm count, while the amino acid carnitine is said to affect sperm motility. *Zinc* has been found to be low in some couples suffering from infertility. But a word of warning: too much zinc can suppress your immune system, according to a report in the *Journal of Alternative Medicine*, August 1986. As always you should only take supplements under the supervision of a nutritional practitioner.

Sitz baths

Cold sitz baths may aid poor sperm production.

Homeopathy/herbalism

Where infertility is associated with adhesions in the internal organs, a homeopathic/herbal approach is sometimes successful. An alternative practitioner who is also medically qualified warns that couples shouldn't pin all their hopes on such methods. "If they are going to work, they will usually have done so by three to six months of treatment," he says.

Hormone problems can be treated by an approach in which homeopathic dosages of progesterone and estrogen are given. The herb, *Vitex agnus castus*, chaste-berry, is especially useful for helping rebalance hormone levels where this is a problem. A medical herbalist comments that herbal treatment can be very successful in cases of hostile mucus.

Acupuncture

Ear acupuncture can often make a significant contribution where the menstrual cycle is irregular. One South African gynecologist in a small-scale study of fifteen to twenty patients found that 60 percent got pregnant within three months by using this method.

The practitioner I mentioned earlier warns: "Infertility is an extremely complex subject and requires someone who understands both complementary and orthodox methods. Unfortunately, these are few and far between." When should you give up? This practitioner says: "It's a difficult question and there are no clear rules; a lot depends on age. I'm very much against people being conned when there is no hope. I'd say after six to nine months of treatment you should think carefully about whether or not to continue."

Finally, before leaving the subject of infertility, here are some anecdotal reports culled from the pages of the National Association for the Childless newsletter in England: "I overcame my fertility problems, investigated but not conclusive, with acupuncture. In early pregnancy I was taught self-hypnosis and have to date had three sessions. I have found it to be of tremendous help in that it has given me confidence."

Another writer describing long-standing problems with ovarian cysts and blocked fallopian tubes says: "I began acupuncture treatments, thinking it might help me to relax if nothing else. I also took Clomiphere for one cycle. One month later I was pregnant! It would seem to be a combination of factors which did the trick. A sympathetic, caring consultant and the encouragement of a skilled acupuncturist, advice on diet and stress (I previously drank up to six cups of coffee daily) and just the knowledge that my perseverance and decisive action were getting me somewhere—all played their part."

She adds: "You must not give up until you have explored areas such as acupuncture and homeopathy. These treatments can be complementary to whatever medical treatment is being received."

Finally, a carroty tale: "After three years of infertility tests, no treatment and no joy, we had given up any hope of having a baby. My husband had a very low sperm count and poor motility...I read about the carrot diet and decided to feed my husband carrots with most meals. This was last May. In July I was pregnant. Whether the carrots had anything to do with our success we shall never know. But to any couples with the same problem as ours, I would say it is worth a try."

For further information:

Resolve Inc.
5 Water St.
Arlington, MA 02174
(617) 643-2424

Infertility—A Common-Sense Guide for the Childless, Andrew Stanway (Thorsons).

Pre-conceptional Care

The idea of encouraging women and men to lead a healthy life before pregnancy has hit the headlines in the last few years. There's a fair body of evidence to suggest that getting fit and well before conception can help avoid some problems later in pregnancy. The incidence of spina bifida and similar defects, for instance, has been shown in trials to be reduced in women taking a vitamin and mineral supplement before pregnancy. And certainly no one would argue with the advice to avoid nonessential prescription and over-the-counter drugs. But a large number of alternative practitioners go one step further.

Far too many women, they argue, enter pregnancy mildly malnourished. The Pill disturbs the metabolism and alters the balance of nutrients in the body. They may have been living on a diet of convenience foods and restaurant meals. And they may be suffering from allergies or minor infections such as cystitis or yeast, which can impair the body's ability to absorb food or deplete it of certain nutrients.

In addition, some women are overweight or have been dieting. Add the well-publicized dangers of smoking, drinking, and environmental pollutants, all of which are known—at least to some extent—to cross the placenta and, claim these experts, you have potential for disaster. "A woman may be healthy enough for all normal purposes but when it comes to taking on the additional burden of pregnancy and feeding another human being it may be different," says a clinical ecologist working in the field.

So what should you make of it all? By all means try to get yourself fit and well before getting pregnant. Having a physical, routine blood chemistries, and a complete blood count is a good idea. But ordinary common-sense measures such as those given in Part One are probably sufficient to ensure that you are in good health. It's also sensible to make sure you haven't any lurking infections such as yeast or cystitis, and the alternative approaches described earlier can help here.

Most women do best taking a prenatal multivitamin/mineral supplement to ensure getting enough of some vitamins and minerals needed in extra amounts by pregnant and nursing women. Pregnant women need 1,200 mg of calcium, 500 mg of magnesium, and 800 mcg of folic acid a day, in addition to slightly higher amounts of iron, zinc, iodine, and vitamins A, E, C, and B complex than they do when they are not pregnant. A good diet may provide all your vitamin and mineral needs during pregnancy, but it doesn't hurt to take a supplement to be sure. If you've previously given birth to a handicapped baby, it may be worth consulting a practitioner interested in nutritional methods

before getting pregnant, in case other specific vitamin/mineral supplementation is needed. However, the chances are that even if you don't do any of these
things you'll have a perfectly healthy baby. And it could be argued that stress
reduction is equally important in the prevention of prematurity and low birth
weight as any other sort of treatment.

Having a Healthy Pregnancy

The secret of having a healthy pregnancy is to pay special attention to the
areas of your life outlined in Part One. Eat a good whole food diet, get enough
exercise and relaxation, and cut stress to the minimum. There are lots of new
things going on in your life when you are pregnant, and a whole different set
of circumstances to adjust to. The growth of a new life inside you may make
you especially open to the spiritual side of life. Many women find meditation
and guided fantasy work especially creative and uplifting when they are pregnant.

✍ What should I eat?

By and large, the rules for healthy eating are the same during pregnancy as
at any other time. Concentrate on getting fresh, good quality foods, choosing
a few foods from the following four food groups.

1. *Dairy products*—milk, yogurt, cheese. If you are allergic or intolerant to
these, you should avoid dairy products and supplement your diet with calcium
and magnesium.

2. *Proteins*—nuts, beans, seeds, meat, fish, and eggs.

3. *Vegetables and fruit*—green leafy vegetables, dried fruits, any other fruit and
vegetables in season, juices.

4. *Bread and cereals*—brown rice and other whole grains, muesli, oatmeal,
whole-grain bread, whole-wheat or rye crispbread.

At one time there were strict limits placed on how much weight women
were supposed to gain in pregnancy. Today this is much more flexible. Unless you are very overweight it's undesirable to diet when you are pregnant.
On the other hand, don't go hog wild and gain fifty pounds or more. For
an average-size woman going into pregnancy at a normal weight, any gain
above thirty-five pounds is going to be excess weight that will not improve
fetal health, and will most likely be difficult to lose after the birth. Besides,
being very overweight at term increases the tendency to tearing during
delivery, and the possibility of excessive postpartum blood loss. If you do

need to lose weight it's best to do it under supervision, so ask your midwife or a qualified practitioner interested in nutritional methods.

There's some evidence to show that if you are very underweight when you start pregnancy, you are more at risk of giving birth to a low birth weight baby. The answer is to use the stress relieving measures outlined in Part One, and eat a good diet of the type described above and elsewhere.

As for eating for two, not many of us believe you have to do that nowadays. In fact, if you did, you would probably end up vastly overweight. Recent studies suggest that the recommended level of 2,400 calories a day for pregnant women might be too high. Women in the study whose average food intakes were 2,000 to 2,200 calories produced perfectly healthy babies, and the premature birth rate was lower than expected.

✍ Minor ailments of pregnancy

Pregnancy is not an illness. Even so, many women are plagued by a number of irritating minor ailments. It's best to avoid taking any drugs unless they are prescribed by your doctor during pregnancy, and this is where alternative remedies can be so helpful.

Morning sickness

About half of all women suffer some degree of nausea or vomiting in early pregnancy. It's thought to be due to increased levels of the human hormone chorionic gonadotrophin (CG), which is produced early on in pregnancy. In very severe cases (hyperemesis), there may be a psychological component, in which case any of the mind-body therapies may be especially useful if you want to avoid hospital admission.

Herbal remedies—for morning sickness include chamomile or peppermint tea. Ginger—either a quarter of an ounce of crystallized or grated root ginger added to a cup of boiling water with honey to taste, or a teaspoon of dried ginger—may be helpful too.

Homeopathic remedies—also useful for morning sickness. Self-help homeopathic remedies are best taken in the sixth potency; if these aren't effective, see a qualified homeopath to see whether a more powerful potency is recommended. The following, quoted in *Birth Matters*, edited by Ros Claxton (Unwin Paperbacks), are especially useful:

♂ *Ipecacuanha*—if you feel irritable and resentful about the pregnancy.

♂ *Phosphorus*—you are indifferent but crave sympathy. You are anxious about others and afraid of being on your own. You crave fresh air and cold drinks, but may be sick after them.

♂ *Sepia*—if you feel indifferent toward those you love, are depressed, and can't stand noise and smells.

♂ *Pulsatilla*—you weep easily, are moody, and crave sympathy.

♂ *Ignatia*—you do unexpected irrational things.

♂ *Aurum*—if you are deeply depressed.

Diet—may also play a part in helping to avoid morning sickness. Eat small, regular meals. These are some other tricks worth trying: Avoid highly spiced or fatty foods. Have milky drinks and soup if you can't keep anything down. Drink mineral waters and fruit juices rather than tea and coffee, which can increase nausea. Keep a hoard of snacks to nibble on during the day.

Rest—get regular rest periods during the day. See if you can arrange with your boss to go in a bit later to avoid the rush hour. Try to get one or two early nights a week. Avoid nonessential housework.

Supplements—Vitamin B_6 seems to help some women. Take 50-200 mg a day. Zinc is also useful; try 25-50 mg a day. Some women find that taking betaine HCl, a tablet form of hydrochloric acid, with protein meals is very helpful in relieving morning sickness. Stomach production of hydrochloric acid is often depressed in early pregnancy and taking a little extra can improve digestion and relieve queasiness. Signs that you may need extra hydrochloric acid are bloating and queasiness after eating protein foods, and cravings for sour foods such as pickles. It is usually best to start with one five-grain tablet with the meal. If this causes more discomfort, do not take any more and eat some protein to use up the acid. If it doesn't help but doesn't cause problems either, you may increase the number of pills until you see results. At any rate, don't go above four pills per meal without your doctor's OK, and only take them with protein meals; stop them entirely if you experience heartburn or other discomfort. You shouldn't need to take them at all after the third month of pregnancy. It is advisable to consult a qualified nutritional practitioner for further suggestions.

Severe sickness—lie down and keep perfectly still with a hot water bottle over your abdomen. Hang in there—it'll soon be over. Most cases of morning sickness wear off by twelve to sixteen weeks into the pregnancy.

Heartburn

Generally this is more of a problem during the later weeks of pregnancy. Lying semi-propped up in bed and having a milk drink at bedtime can help. Liquid calcium/magnesium supplements—one to two teaspoons at a time up to twelve teaspoons a day—can help neutralize the acid. Herbal remedies include meadowsweet made up as a tea and sipped on and off during the day. Aniseed, with mint or lavender added, or a combination of powdered slippery elm and marshmallow root, one-half teaspoon at a time, may also be helpful. For further advice consult an herbal practitioner. Avoid eating over-spiced foods and eat little and often.

Constipation

This is sometimes a problem during pregnancy because of the relaxing effects of circulating hormones on smooth muscle. The answer is to make sure you have a good whole-grain diet, with plenty of raw foods. Drink plenty of fluids. Lemon juice in hot water on rising is a good trick to try. Herbal remedies may help, but as it's wise to avoid any drugs, including laxatives, during pregnancy you should consult an herbal practitioner to make sure it is safe. Powdered psyllium hull preparations such as Metamucil, however, can be safely used during pregnancy. Recommended dosage is one rounded teaspoon in a full glass of water followed within one hour by another glass of liquid. This can be taken once or twice a day. A tip recommended in an article by antenatal teacher Liz Winkler in *Parents* magazine is to take half a dessertspoonful of linseed in a glass of lukewarm water. She also recommends yoga (see below). Drink two glasses of water and rest in the frog position for ten minutes.

Insomnia

This can be because of anxiety over the pregnancy, or simply because your increased bulk makes it difficult to get comfortable. Homeopathic remedies include arnica, nux vomica, carbo vegetabilis, aurum, and ignatia. For further details consult a homeopath. Aromatherapy may be helpful. Sprinkle one or two drops of oil of lavender, chamomile, marjoram, or clary sage in your bath. Better still, get your partner to give you a massage with warm oils—and sprinkle a few drops of one of the oils on your pillow at night.

Hemorrhoids

You are less likely to get these if you are following the whole food diet recommended. Sponging them with ice-cold water will bring relief, as will sitting in a cold sitz bath. Itching can be relieved by bathing the hemorrhoids in an infusion of witch hazel. Keep your stools soft to avoid straining, and use moistened tissue after moving your bowels. Blot, don't wipe. Then apply either petroleum jelly or an herbal hemorrhoid ointment and gently push any protruding hemorrhoids back inside the rectum. Cold witch hazel compresses can give a lot of relief. Another home remedy which works well for some is to dip a peeled clove of garlic, pricked all over with a pin to release the juices, in honey and insert it rectally after each bowel movement. It's best not to take herbs internally unless recommended by a qualified practitioner.

Yoga poses such as the fish, plough, and shoulder stand can all help hemorrhoids. Homeopathic remedies include calcarea fluorica (for bleeding and itching), hamamelis (when oozing dark blood), ignatia for painful protruding (hemorrhoids), and for itching again, nux vomica.

Varicose veins

Some women develop varicose veins for the first time in pregnancy. Taking plenty of exercise, wearing special support tights, and sitting with your feet raised can all help. Much of the advice applying to hemorrhoids, especially exercising, is useful here. A handful of dried marigold flowers steeped in a cup of witch hazel, then applied to each leg with cloths can bring relief, as will handbaths containing a mixture of hawthorn, broom flowers, yarrow, and rose petals. For internal remedies, consult a qualified herbalist.

Homeopathic remedies include hamamelis in tincture form, carbo vegetabilis to improve circulation, and after you've had the baby, pulsatilla.

High blood pressure

Very high blood pressure (over 140/90), especially if combined with protein in your urine, swelling, eyesight problems or headaches, needs medical attention either from an orthodox doctor or a medically qualified alternative practitioner. However, less severe blood pressure problems can be successfully treated by using relaxation techniques. In one study, meditation combined with biofeedback was found to be successful in avoiding the need for hospital admission and bedrest in a group of women with mild high blood pressure. Another way of reducing elevated blood pressure, when stress induced, is to consciously tense every muscle group in your body for two or three seconds, then relax. This seems to help the muscles relax more completely, and lowers blood pressure. It can be repeated many times a day if necessary.

High blood pressure can be treated by cutting out tea and coffee and substituting an herb tea such as lime blossom instead. Taking garlic either in capsule form or by eating three or four medium cloves a day will help reduce blood pressure. Also, dandelion greens and roots can be used to help reduce water retention, which in turn affects blood pressure. Check with an herbalist or naturopath for dosage. Footbaths of hawthorn, celandine, and broom flowers with a head of garlic are recommended in *The Alternative Directory of Symptoms and Cures*, by Caroline Shreeve (Century). Homeopathy can also be useful, as can reflexology.

Pre-eclamptic toxemia

This is a condition of pregnancy involving the three symptoms of high blood pressure, swelling, and protein in the urine. The Brewer diet, outlined below, is a high calorie diet devised by American nutritionist Tom Brewer and is said to prevent pre-eclamptic toxemia.

Each day:

4 glasses milk (2 pints)	grapefruit, tomato, large glass fresh fruit juice
2 eggs	
3 servings fish, shelffish, turkey/chicken (4 ounces per serving)	3 pats butter
	5 yellow or orange fruits or vegetables per week
2 helpings of fresh, green leafy vegetables	
	Liver once a week
5 servings bread, pasta, whole grain cereal, brown rice	Salt to taste
2 choices from whole potato, lemon,	Fluids to taste

Follow the stress-relieving measures described in Part One, and pay attention to getting a good night's sleep.

Stretch marks

There's no sure way to avoid stretch marks, though not gaining too much weight and making sure you are not overweight to start with may help. Some women have said the following remedy helps: 2 dessert-spoonsful of wheat germ oil added to a teaspoon of lavender oil in a cup of almond oil, massaged in every day. A cream or ointment containing vitamin E can be used the same way. Taking extra vitamin E, 200-400 IU a day, and 30-50 mg of zinc a day has helped some women.

Acupuncture for pregnancy and childbirth

Acupuncture can tune up your body so that it is in the best possible shape to cope with pregnancy and childbirth; it makes a useful adjunct to the types of pre-pregnancy care mentioned earlier. It can also help with morning sickness, urinary problems, high blood pressure, swelling, and fatigue. In the book *Birth Matters*, edited by Ros Claxton, natural healer Carol Rudd claims that acupuncture can be used to turn a baby from a wrong position, and during birth if the placenta fails to come away or if you develop postpartum hemorrhage (bleeding). This could be due to the effect acupuncture has on uterine contractions. A study carried out by a medical student under the auspices of the Centre for the Study of Alternative Therapies looked at the possibility of inducing labor by using electroacupuncture. In fact, only one woman went into labor with acupuncture alone. However, acupuncture did seem to increase the number and strength of contractions. Further studies are obviously needed to see how useful it might in fact be.

Yoga and pregnancy

Yoga is a particularly appropriate form of antenatal preparation, joining as it does body, mind, and spirit. Many women are now seeking out yoga preparation for childbirth as an alternative to more traditional types of relaxation and breathing classes. And yoga plays an important part in many of the "alternative" birth classes.

It's a big subject, and if you are interested in finding out more, I'd advise you to read *Yoga in Pregnancy* by Vibeke Borg (Watkins). Here I'll just outline a few of the benefits to be gained from regular yoga practice during pregnancy. On the following pages you'll see illustrated a few of the postures that might be especially useful.

Physical benefits

It helps you develop a strong supple body and back, so that you can bear the stresses and strains of pregnancy more easily. It helps with posture and so may alleviate backache and other aches and pains. It strengthens the body without tightening the muscles—this is important for birth.

Breathing

Breath control exercises improve the oxygen flow in your blood and to and from the placenta. Learning to control your breathing is especially useful during labor. You can breathe more deeply or lightly to reduce pain from contractions and help you deal with pain. Smooth, calm breathing helps you relax and relieves anxiety.

Mental benefits

Concentration and meditation can help you to focus in on yourself, a useful skill during labor when the sensations from the uterus can be overwhelming. This again can help with pain relief. More important, yoga can help you have confidence in the way your body operates, so that you are less likely to get frightened during labor. Experts have pointed to a strong connection between fear, tension, and pain in labor. If you practice yoga regularly, you'll be able to listen to your body and know instinctively what postures are most likely to help you during labor.

After you have had your baby, yoga can help relax you, and can give you a calm center in a life that has probably drastically changed. Sophy Hoare says in *Birth Matters:*

"To try to hold on to a fixed image of yourself leads to suffering when the image can no longer hold its own against reality; at the same time, behind ideas and images can be found the unchanging centre of the self when we are able to let go of our fixed attitudes and expectations. Yoga brings us in touch with the flow of life and with the enduring centre; in this way changes in our circumstances can be accepted without fear of losing our personal identity."

♫ Osteopathy for pregnancy

Osteopathy can be used in the pre-pregnancy period to help rebalance your body. It's especially useful for the problems caused by the changing weight load of your body, which can cause backache and other aches and pains during pregnancy. Treating the back can increase blood flow to the pelvic area. Osteopathy can also be useful during labor itself; pressure at the base of the spine can help soothe pain, and techniques such as "hanging" from a rope or pole can help stretch the lower part of your spine, which may relieve pain. After birth osteopathy can help realign your pelvis and spine.

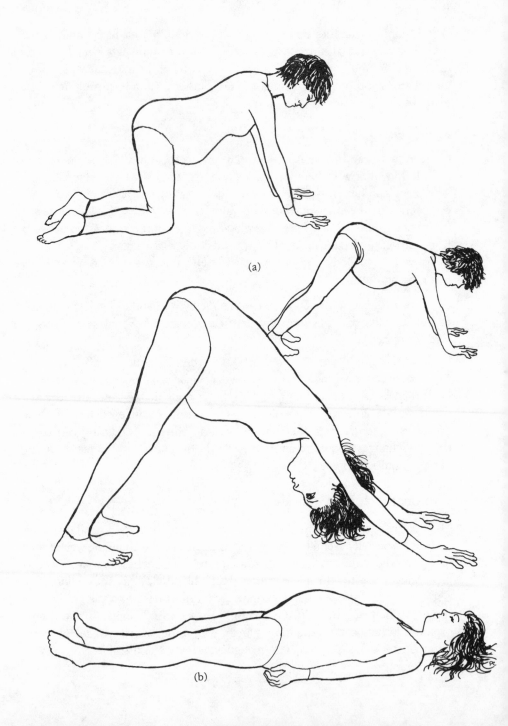

(a)

(b)

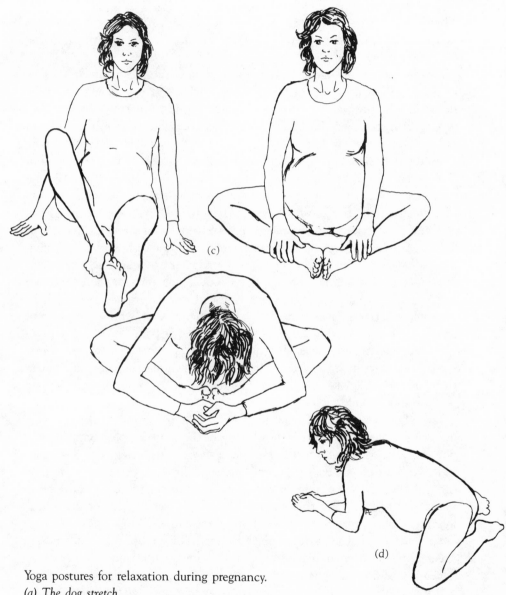

Yoga postures for relaxation during pregnancy.

(a) The dog stretch.

(b) Savasana—the pose for deep relaxation.

(c) The star.

(d) The frog.

Birth—Pain Relief

There's a vast amount written on birth, and there isn't really space here to do the subject full justice, so we plan to concentrate on alternative pain relief for labor.

Most women would agree that labor is painful. Only an estimated 5 percent of us get away with a completely painless birth. And the popular image of the primitive tribeswoman who squats casually and painlessly behind a bush to give birth is fallacy. Orthodox medicine's answer to the problem of pain in labor is to do away with it by giving drugs. Unfortunately, all the pain-relieving drugs used during labor have quite serious disadvantages as you can see from the section on orthodox methods of pain relief (following). At least one prominent obstetrician has expressed the opinion that the disadvantages of Demerol—still the most widely used painkiller in labor—outweigh its advantages. Epidurals can completely relieve pain. But a survey carried out in 1982 at London's Queen Charlotte's Maternity Hospital showed that having an epidural doesn't necessarily guarantee a happier experience in childbirth. In fact, it may do the opposite. Of the 1,000 women studied, those who had received an epidural were more dissatisfied with the experience of childbirth, both immediately afterward and a year later, than women who had refused all analgesia and those who accepted simpler forms of pain relief.

The alternative birth movement that has grown up in the last few years points out that many women could go without pain relief altogether, or could reduce their need for it, if they are allowed to walk around and choose the positions that are most comfortable.

The whole issue of pain relief in labor is a thorny one, because it is tied up with the question of who controls childbirth. Quite simply, giving a pain-relieving drug is something the medical staff can do to help you if you are in labor. You ring the bell for a nurse during labor and the chances are that she will offer you something for the pain. Your fear and need will have been interpreted as pain, and this in turn strengthens the conventional medical interpretation of that need as stemming from pain.

The fact is that pain isn't an objective fact. All sorts of other factors can affect it: being in unfamiliar surroundings, being stranded on your back and forced to stay in the same position because you are wired up to a monitor, and interventions such as acceleration (speeding up) of labor itself can all affect the amount of pain you feel. In Holland, where the majority of births take place at home, only 5 percent of women have pain-relieving drugs, compared with 70-80 percent in this country. Why? Assuming that Dutch women can't be endowed with more courage than we are, it could be that they accept pain as part of the process of giving birth, whereas we are conditioned to believe that all pain should be removed. It could also have a lot to do with the circumstances of birth.

It's known that physical and emotional support during labor can reduce or even eliminate the need for other forms of pain relief, partly because labor is likely to be shorter in these circumstances. Also, the more relaxed you are the more efficiently your uterus operates.

If you feel you would prefer the minimum of drugs and intervention, and as long as your pregnancy is straightforward, it might be worth considering a home delivery or delivery in a midwifery clinic. If you do have to go into the hospital, make sure your wishes are written on your chart. This is where your assertiveness techniques come in too. Many alternative birth teachers offer assertiveness training as part of preparation for birth.

Alternative and self-help approaches to pain relief in labor

Stay up and about

The illustrations here show suitable positions for first- and second-stage labor. The more upright you can be, the stronger contractions are and the more effective, since the baby's descent is aided by gravity. An upright position also improves blood supply to the baby, so the baby is likely to withstand the stress and strain of labor better, and less likely to be short of oxygen (become distressed).

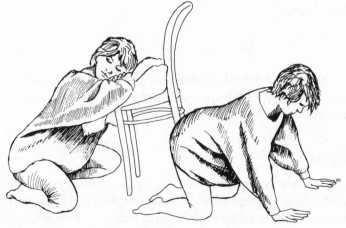

First- and second-stage labor positions.

Relaxation

Make yourself at home if you are going into the hospital. Take in something familiar that you like to look at, such as a picture or a vase of flowers. Having something to concentrate on such as a picture, a candle, or a visual image can also help you focus inward, which in turn helps relieve pain.

Take a companion with you. This could be your partner, a relative, or a friend.

Massage

Massage will help ease pain. Low back massage using a firm circular motion, or getting your partner to roll a tennis ball over your lumbar region is very soothing. Effleurage—light fingertip massage—over your abdomen will be helpful too.

Acupuncture

Acupuncture has been very successfully used to relieve labor pains, and caesarean sections have even been performed using acupuncture as the only anesthetic. If you want to take an acupuncturist into the hospital, it will be necessary to get the permission of your doctor. A pilot study carried out by a midwife in Glasgow and reported in *Midwives Chronicle,* May 1985, found that 75 percent of women in labor who had received acupuncture said they would opt for it again next time they had a baby: "Common comments from the women in the study related to a feeling of 'calmness' and the maintenance of self control during labor."

Hypnosis

Hypnosis helps some women deal with labor pain, perhaps by easing tension. If you want to use hypnotherapy you should start to learn the necessary techniques from early on in pregnancy.

Herbal remedies

These can be extremely effective in toning up your uterus in preparation for labor, so that it is in the best possible shape. Raspberry leaf tea is one of the best known tried-and-tested remedies—you can drink it during the last three months (three heaping teaspoons to a pot of tea taken two to three times a day). However, it is probably best to consult a qualified herbalist before taking it, since raspberry leaves can tone up or relax the uterus. In some very athletic women the muscles of the uterus can become overtoned. Squaw vine (*Mitchella repens*) is another useful remedy, as is blue cohosh (Caulophyllum). You may also want to use aromatherapy oils such as rosemary oil or lavender and chamomile during labor, either rubbed on to your forehead, wrists, and neck or used in massage.

Homeopathic remedies

These include Caulophyllum to tone up the uterus, and arnica which prevents and eases bruising. A homeopath will be able to recommend other suitable remedies tailored to you as an individual for use during labor itself.

Hot baths

A hot bath can be extremely helpful in relieving pain and promoting relaxation during labor. In first stage labor, they can increase the speed of cervical dilation and can greatly improve comfort; in fact, some women don't want to get out when it's time for the actual delivery!

TENS

Transcutaneous electrical nerve stimulation is an offshoot of acupuncture, and some acupuncturists believe it offers better pain relief than traditional acupuncture techniques, especially as some women dislike having the needles inserted during labor. Another advantage is that an increasing number of hospitals now have TENS equipment. TENS works by sending electrical impulses to the brain; these impulses block pain messages and stimulate the release of endorphins (the body's own pain-relieving hormones). Incidentally, this may be the key to how many alternative pain-relief methods work. The equipment consists of a small hand-held box with four electrodes which can be placed on particular acupunture points on your back or abdomen. The sensation is one of vibration or pins and needles, which changes to a continuous electrical sensation. It's thought that TENS is successful in wiping out about 95 percent of back pain during labor. And one midwife we spoke to reported that it could help some women to manage entirely without pain-relieving drugs. Others might need some pain relief as a back up. But as one of a battery of other methods, TENS certainly seems worth a try.

⌗ Orthodox methods of pain relief

Demerol

Still the most widely used drug for pain relief, although it has been somewhat replaced in recent years by the epidural. It's given by injection. At its best it may make you feel relaxed and slightly woozy. But many women complain that it makes them feel drunk and out of control. It can also make you sick. The main disadvantage is that it crosses the placenta, and babies exposed to large quantities tend to be drowsier and slower to suck. Some babies suffer breathing difficulties, so another drug which reverses the effects of Demerol has to be given. In one study, mothers who had had large doses of Demerol spent less time looking after and holding their babies in the hour after birth than did a control group. This could be due to the distancing effect of the drug, though it could also be argued that someone who had needed large amounts of Demerol might have had a pretty lousy labor anyway, and just wanted to rest after it all.

Epidural

The only pain-relieving procedure that can completely remove pain. It causes complete lack of sensation from the abdomen downward, which some women find unpleasant. Drawbacks include the fact that once the epidural is in place (the drug is inserted via a catheter into the epidural space in your spine), you can no longer move around. What's more, if you have an epidural you'll be far more likely to have a very medically managed labor. You'll need to be electronically monitored since you won't be able to feel contractions. You may also need forceps delivery because unless the epidural is timed to wear off, you won't be able to feel the pushing sensations of second-stage labor. Because of the paralysis of your pelvic floor muscles, the baby's head often doesn't rotate as it should—hence the need for forceps.

Paracervical block

Used in first-stage labor, this consists of the infiltration of a local anesthetic on either side of the cervix. It reduces pain from cervical stretching without affecting other sensations or uterine contractions. It produces transient slowing of the baby's heart beat in 30 percent of cases. A few women have severe sensitivity reactions to local anesthetics.

Gas and air

Perhaps the most acceptable of orthodox pain-relieving methods. It's a mixture of nitrous oxide (laughing gas) and oxygen which you breathe in at the start of each contraction. Pain relief is good, and because the gas passes out of your body between contractions there is less danger that it will pass into your baby's system in large amounts. It seems to have less effect on the baby than Demerol, and the level in your baby's blood falls rapidly as breathing begins.

After the Birth—Getting Back to Normal

◌ Stitches

If you've had stitches, the following alternative remedies are useful:

Arnica for bruising. Take internally in homeopathic dosage.

◌ Aim a warm hair dryer at the sore area.

◌ Cold ice packs against the stitches.

◌ Do your pelvic floor exercises to stimulate circulation to the area; this aids healing.

◌ Apply witch hazel and mix it with three parts water to soothe soreness.

◌ Calendula ointment can help too.

◌ Breast-feeding

Success in breast-feeding depends on being able to feed your baby whenever the baby feels hungry, coupled with a good diet, sufficient rest, and a large dose of confidence. Probably more women give up on breast-feeding through lack of advice and support than for any other reason. However, there are one or two specific problems that can be overcome by using a combination of self help and alternative techniques.

Insufficient milk supply

This is probably the most common reason women give up breast-feeding. Make sure you are eating a good whole food diet, with plenty of fluids. Have mineral water and fruit juices. Probably apple and grape are best, as orange juice seems to disagree with some babies and make them colicky. Feed frequently. Milk supply relies on frequent stimulation of the nipples, which stimulates hormones to send messages to the breasts to produce more milk. Goat's rue (*Galega officinale*) (one or two tablespoonfuls to a cup) made into a tea is a useful herbal remedy. Take it three times a day. For other remedies consult a qualified herbalist. Tension can interfere with your milk supply by inhibiting the "let down reflex," which makes the milk flow out of your nipples and send messages to the breasts to produce more milk. Relaxation, yoga, and meditation can all be good ways of relieving tension. There are numerous homeopathic remedies to increase milk supply—these include *Vitex agnus castus*, asafoetida, causticum, pulsatilla, and urtica urens. Consult a homeopath for further advice.

Sore nipples

As well as being unpleasant in themselves, sore nipples can inhibit the milk supply by making you tense. Make sure your baby is properly positioned at the breast. The whole of the nipple and the brown area (areola) around it should be in the baby's mouth, and the nipple should be well back in the mouth so it is not pressing on the hard palate. If your nipples do get sore, start the feeding on the less sore side first. Expose your nipples to the air as much as you can. The air jet from a warm hair dryer or convection heater will aid healing. Allow a drop of breast milk to dry on the nipples—it contains a substance that helps healing. Bag Balm or calendula ointment can be used. Homeopathic remedies include the good old faithful arnica, calendula as an ointment and/or taken internally, castor equi., graphites, and chamomilla to mention a few. Consult a homeopath for other ideas.

For further information on breast-feeding, contact:

> La Leche League International
> Box 1209-9616 Minneapolis Ave.
> Franklin Park, IL
> (312) 455-7730

Postnatal depression

One study suggests that nearly 40 percent of women suffer postnatal depression. More conservative estimates put the figure at 10-15 percent. Even if they don't develop full-blown depression, many women complain of chronic tiredness, and other niggling aches and pains such as backache, headaches, hemorrhoids, menstrual pains, and coughs and colds—all of which have been associated with depression and certainly do nothing for mental well-being.

It's all a far cry from the rosy picture of motherhood that we get from the ad-men. The snag is that even the experts haven't decided among themselves just what causes postnatal depression. Is it a true depressive illness? Is it triggered by the hormonal upheavals of pregnancy and birth? Or does it arise out of the conditions of motherhood—the lack of recognition, isolation, and so on, that go hand in hand with being a mother in our society? On the one hand we're told it's the most important job in the world, but all the "rewards" which are traditionally allotted to valued jobs, such as high pay, status, and all the rest are noticeably missing. Vivienne Welburn, author of *Postnatal Depression* (Fontana), who has herself suffered from it, said:

"Postnatal depression is a result of all sorts of factors. Women are highly vulnerable and sensitive after having a baby and things affect them more than they would normally."

In psychological terms, childbirth has been described as a "crisis"—a major life event, which requires an enormous amount of readjustment. An Australian midwife and anthropologist speaking at the 1986 Marce Society conference pointed out that in closer-knit rural communities in undeveloped parts of the world, postnatal depression is unknown.

Orthodox treatment consists of anti-depressant drugs, hormones (Dr. Katharina Dalton, whose work on premenstrual tension we described earlier, is the major proponent of this theory), and occasionally psychotherapy. The latest research is aimed at discovering which women are vulnerable to postnatal depression, with a view to intervening by offering extra support and counseling.

What are the signs of postnatal depression?

Postnatal depression is different from fourth day "blues," which most of us experience just after birth, and which does appear to have a strong hormonal component. In fact, depression may not be the main symptom at all. An unnatural high or excessive anxiety are both common. Postnatal depression sufferers will suffer some or more of the following: sadness, lack of self-esteem, loss of interest in former pleasures (such as food, sex, clothes), weepiness, despair, guilt, self reproach, exhaustion, irritability, inability to cope, feelings of isolation, and withdrawal. You may experience fears connected with your baby's welfare, or alternatively be frightened that you are going to harm the baby.

Alternative treatments

Diet

Some interesting new research from the Department of Child Health at the Hospital for Sick Children in Bristol, England, has looked at levels of vitamins B_2 (riboflavin) and B_6 (pyridoxine) in a group of twenty mothers suffering from postnatal illness. Half the depressed group were found to be lacking in B_2, and the depressed group had lower B_6 levels than a control group. Antibiotics and smoking have a marked effect on the levels of these vitamins.

Given that vitamin B_6 is especially susceptible to the effects of processing, it could be that many mothers who are depressed are simply not getting enough vitamins in their diet. The researchers also comment that "more attention could be paid in this country to rebalancing vitamin levels and restoring gut flora after antibiotic treatment." But they also suggest that the low vitamin levels could be a reflection of poor appetite in the depressed group. It looks as though it would be worth seeing a practitioner interested in nutrition before deciding to take antidepressants.

Herbalism and Homeopathy

Many of the therapies suggested in the section on mental health are equally applicable to postnatal depression. Herbal treatments seem to work very well, with the emphasis being put on herbs that rebalance and integrate hormonal levels. Herbs such as scullcap and valerian may be used to alleviate depression and anxiety.

There are also a number of homeopathic remedies which could be useful. In his book, *A Woman's Guide to Homeopathic Medicine* (Thorsons), Dr. Trevor Smith suggests a number of useful remedies, of which he says sepia is the most useful and should be tried first. The profile is "weakness, sadness, and tiredness. A sense of indifference to everything and everybody is marked, together with obstinate constipation, constant hunger, and a yellowish-brown facial discoloration." For further details of the remedy that is right for you consult a homeopath.

Finally, osteopathy seems to be useful in some cases of postnatal depression.

Menopause

Menopause simply means the end of your periods. It can start as early as your thirties or as late as your sixties. It can also happen if for any reason you have to have your ovaries removed (oophorectomy). For most women, it occurs between the ages of forty-five and fifty-five.

Like so many of the other conditions described in this book, menopause is surrounded by myths. Like premenstrual syndrome and childbirth, the problems many of us experience during the menopause are seen and treated as medical ones, when perhaps they can be better understood in relation to all the other things going on in our lives at the time. Menopause, for instance, often coincides with children leaving home, the loss of parents or a spouse through divorce or death, or the onset of ill health, all of which can cause stress. And as we've seen time and again now, stress can affect you and make any pre-existing symptoms worse. What's more, living in a culture where young is beautiful, and older women are considered over the hill sexually, can be enough to provoke depression and lack of self-esteem.

☞ What signs and symptoms are associated with menopause?

The catalog of complaints makes depressing reading: vaginal dryness, hot flashes, night sweats, painful sex, dry skin, cramps, varicose veins, sore breasts, aches and pains in the joints, anxiety, depression, and brittle bones are the main ones. But even so, only some 10 percent of women suffer really disabling symptoms according to the statistics, and chances are you might only experience one or two of these. Fortunately, there are a lot of things you can do to help yourself.

☞ Orthodox treatment

The familiar gamut of hormone treatment, tranquilizers, and antidepressants is orthodox medicine's answer to the problems of menopause.

Hormone replacement therapy (HRT) is often prescribed, especially if you are troubled by hot flashes, the idea being that it is lack of estrogen that causes flushing and vaginal changes. HRT is taken in pill form, rather like the contraceptive pill. It consists of estrogen with, nowadays, progestin added, which means that you will get an artificial period every month. The snag is that we don't really know whether it is actually lack of estrogen that causes the flashes. What's more, there is disturbing evidence that HRT leads to increased incidence of cancer of the uterus and gall bladder problems. And we still have no idea of its long-term effects. You shouldn't have HRT if you suffer from liver problems, gall bladder disease, certain blood and circulatory disorders, fibroids, or diabetes. And no doctor should prescribe it if you have a family history of breast cancer or cancer of the uterus. Even if you do decide to opt for HRT, don't expect it to work miracles, and try to take the smallest possible dose for the shortest time possible.

♂ Alternative therapies and self help

Flashes and dry vagina

As you'd expect, a good whole food diet is the basis of an alternative approach. Some naturopaths recommend various supplements.

Vitamin E can help an itchy, dry vagina and hot flashes. Doses of between 200 and 600 IU a day are recommended. Experiment to find the lowest level that suits you. If it doesn't work right away, don't give up—it can take three to four weeks to have an effect. Adding vitamins C and the B complex, and gingseng, seems to improve its action. Vitamin E can also be diluted with olive oil and massaged into the vulvar and vaginal tissues once a day. This has helped many women who had vaginal dryness and discomfort in intercourse due to thinning of these tissues after menopause.

A special mention should be made here of *ginseng*, an herb which contans a number of substances that control the hormone levels in your body. In one Finnish study, doctors found it helped dry vagina, hot flashes, sweats, tension, anxiety, and palpitations. Take 600 mg to 1,200 mg a day. It would probably be a good idea to consult an herbal practitioner since the quality of ginseng sold in health food stores varies a lot. Don Quai, another Chinese herb, also has an estrogenic effect and can be used similarly to ginseng, but it should be used under the direction of an herbalist. Also included in *herbal remedies* are the familiar raspberry leaf tea, cramp bark, black cohosh, licorice, and golden seal. Passiflora tablets are useful if you are tense or anxious.

Vitamin F, found in cold-pressed oils such as olive oil, sunflower oil, and linseed oil, is said to help with skin problems and nervousness. Evening primrose oil may also help. Rina Nissim, in *Natural Healing in Gynaecology* (Pandora), recommends supplements of calcium, magnesium, iron, and phosphorus. See the listing on pages 13-17 for naturally occurring forms of these. See a nutritional therapist for further advice. Exercise will help build up your bones and keep you supple. Swimming is a good exercise, as are walking and yoga. The pelvic floor exercises described in Part One can help prevent prolapse and stress incontinence.

Regular sex, either with a partner or by masturbation, is one of the best treatments and is preventive of menopausal problems, especially for lack of elasticity and dryness of the vagina. It also helps reduce stress. So go ahead and enjoy yourself! Aloe vera gel will lubricate your vagina if you have a tendency toward dryness.

Homeopathy can be very helpful in reducing the number and intensity of hot flashes, as well as many other discomforts associated with menopause. Some of the more useful remedies are lachesis, sanguinaria, glonoinum, and sepia, although you will get best results by consulting a homeopathic practitioner.

How to cope with hot flashes

☞ Follow the stress-relieving measures suggested elsewhere in the book.

☞ Cool down with an ice pack, iced water, or freshen-up tissues.

☞ Avoid hot curries and too much spicy food.

☞ Cut out tea, coffee, alcohol, smoking, and too much sugar.

☞ Wear cotton underwear and clothing and use cotton bedsheets to absorb sweat and make you feel more comfortable.

☞ Wear layers of clothing so you can strip down if you feel a flash coming on.

Osteoporosis (brittle bones)

Men and women experience bone loss from their late thirties onward, but women, especially white, small-boned women who live in northern parts of the world, are especially susceptible. Such women have less bone mass to start with. What's more, women tend to get less exercise than men. Exercise can significantly reduce bone loss, according to one study—which is one good reason to start exercising. After menopause, estrogen secretion decreases and bone loss accelerates. Something like five out of ten women will suffer osteoporosis after the age of sixty-five, and a few will suffer very severely. Osteoporosis is responsible for the traditional dowager's hump and the hip fractures that some older women seem prey to. Such problems can be prevented to some extent by getting plenty of calcium with vitamin D to aid absorption. There's evidence too that moderate weight-bearing exercise can be helpful. Experts say we need 700 to 1,000 mg of calcium per day before menopause, and 1,000 to 1,500 mg thereafter. Vitamin D supplements aren't recommended for white women because they are more susceptible to overdosing, except under the supervision of a qualified practitioner.

Making the best of calcium in your diet

Eat a high-fiber diet, but avoid adding extra bran since it contains phytic acid, which can prevent calcium absorption. Alcohol, too, can interfere with calcium metabolism. Too much caffeine and salt can cause it to be excreted. Calcium lactate, gluconate, citrate, and aspartate are good sources of calcium. But, be warned—excess calcium can alter zinc, magnesium and manganese levels in the body, which can cause kidney stones. One rule to follow is to always take at least half as much magnesium as calcium. Some women need closer to a one-to-one ratio. It's best, as with all supplementation, to seek the advice of a practitioner.

Hysterectomy

Although hysterectomies are performed on younger women, you're most likely to be advised to have one if you are older. Hang on to your womb if you possibly can.

Good reasons to have a hysterectomy

🖙 cancer of the cervix or lining of the womb

🖙 large fibroids

🖙 endometriosis or heavy persistent bleeding for any other cause

🖙 disease of the ovaries and fallopian tubes

🖙 cancer of the uterus

🖙 very occasionally, complications of childbirth

(a)

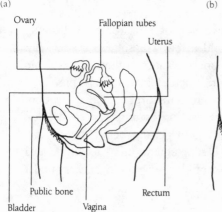

Ovary Fallopian tubes Uterus
Public bone Rectum
Bladder Vagina

(b)

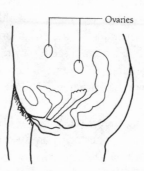

Ovaries

(c)

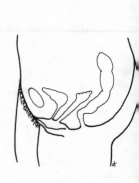

Hysterectomy.
(a) Position of organs before hysterectomy.
(b) Removal of the uterus leaving the ovaries intact.
(c) Removal of the uterus and ovaries.

Decision time

If you're advised to have a hysterectomy, discuss it very carefully with your doctor to ensure that it really is necessary. After the operation you may experience vaginal dryness, and will need time to recover. Not surprisingly, many women get depressed at the loss of their wombs. Acupuncture, reflexology, massage, and homeopathic and herbal remedies may all be helpful in the recovery period. You may also benefit from counseling or psychotherapy to help you come to terms with the operation. Any of the hands-on therapies or healing may be especially useful. A writer in *Nursing Mirror*, May 1985, describes how healing was stimulated by a nurse who held her head and put ice packs on it: "It may sound far-fetched, but I felt something in me respond to her touch, something which in the midst of all the pain, sweat, and tears was the awakening of the will to recover."

For further information, contact:

> The Hysterectomy Education Resource Service (HERS)
> 422 Bryn Mawr
> Bala Cynwyd, PA 19004
> (215) 667-7757

The Therapies

Introduction

All the alternative therapies attempt to treat you as a whole person, that is, they are "holistic," so any method of classifying them is going to seem a bit artificial. However, it's probably true to say that any therapy will take either the mind, body, or spirit as a starting point, though some approaches, such as yoga, integrate the three so completely effective that it's hard to know which aspect of self it acts on first. As you've read through the book, you've been introduced to the possible effects of various alternative therapies. In this section we'd like to give a more complete description of each of these approaches to wellness. If you feel inclined to try a particular therapy that appeals to you, don't be put off by the fact that it hasn't been recommended for your particular complaint. Your intuition will help you develop a sense for the therapy or combination of therapies that will suit your needs best.

♪ Alternative good, orthodox bad?

Alternative medicine has an appeal for women because it very obviously avoids some of the pitfalls outlined in Part One. In our everyday lives we are used to being compartmentalized and fragmented, and alternative medicine may seem especially useful because it does try to see a person as a whole. An alternative practitioner will want to know all about you, where you live, what sort of foods you eat, the quality of your relationships, all about your work, and the degree of satisfaction you feel with your life.

Just as important, as we've seen throughout the book, the alternative therapies work by stimulating the body toward homeostasis and self healing, rather than by suppressing or removing symptoms. This makes the alternative therapies especially suitable for so many of the conditions that are defined as "illness" by the medical profession, but which in actual fact are an integral part of our lives as women, such as pregnancy, menstruation, and menopause.

153

But that's not to say that orthodox is all bad, or that alternative is bound to be good. Alternative therapies can also be considered complimentary therapies, and may work to expedite the healing process put into motion by a medical doctor.

When deciding to treat a condition by alternative means, you will discover that many alternative practitioners are not covered under standard health insurance policies, and many alternative therapies are not covered regardless of who is providing them. However, don't let this discourage you! A growing number of orthodox medical doctors are employing alternative practitioners as part of their health care team. If you are counting on your insurance to cover your treatment, call them first and see who and what is covered. The fees charged by alternative practitioners vary widely depending on the therapy, the practitioner, and the time he or she spends with you. The most expensive doctor is not always the best, so shop around. If you are so fortunate as to live near a training school for the type of therapy you have in mind, the student clinics usually offer treatment at reduced rates.

Just because a treatment is "alternative" doesn't mean it is necessarily safe, although the majority of them are, in the right hands. There have been horror stories of people becoming seriously ill by following certain rigorous diet schedules, for instance, or by taking too many supplements. However, it's important to keep the dangers in perspective—the orthodox medics are just as guilty, if not more so, of iatrogenic (doctor caused) diseases.

The point is that it's just as important to be as critical of alternative therapies as you would orthodox ones, and to choose your practitioner carefully. Make sure you understand your treatment and why it is being done. After all, you'd expect to know why you were taking a new powerful antibiotic, so why not the same for an herb? The issue of self help comes in here too. It is sometimes practical to treat minor ailments yourself by using alternative methods, and throughout the book we've tried to indicate the sorts of things you can do to help yourself. But, reading some of the books on alternative medicine on the market, you could be forgiven for thinking that you could treat almost any illness yourself by using alternative therapies. Most alternative practitioners have to undergo lengthy training, and it would be just as unwise to think you could treat a complex illness such as cancer or endometriosis yourself, without the guidance of a qualified alternative practitioner, as it would without seeing a conventional doctor.

One of the major criticisms of alternative therapies by orthodox medicine is that they have been insufficently tested. This is sometimes due to the nature of the therapy; it would be very difficult to set up large-scale trials of the effectiveness of a certain homeopathic remedy in treating arthritis, for example. There are a great many people with this problem who have been helped by homeopathy, but since the remedies are matched to the patient, not the disease, only a small number of people in such a trial would benefit from any one remedy selected. Also, there is very little money available for testing alternative treatments, and even fewer researchers who are familiar with both accepted testing techniques and alternative therapies. There has been some increase lately in funding for research in certain areas such as acupuncture, nutrition, herbology, and clinical ecology. Hopefully, this trend will continue. In the meantime, while you may wish to try a therapy even if the AMA claims that it has no scientific basis, you don't want to entirely reject conventional scientific methods either. If it hadn't been for studies and trials, for instance, many women would continue to have radical breast surgery for cancers for which a lumpectomy would have been just as good.

Finding a Therapist

Because the therapies are so diverse and some have no central training regulations as does conventional medicine, it can be difficult to find an alternative practitioner. What should you be looking for? And how can you tell if he or she is any good?

Unfortunately, there are no easy answers to these questions because so much depends on the individual. The advice to find out what works for you can be a costly and time-consuming business. And the advice to go to only a recognized or medically trained therapist is not as simple as it seems on the face of it either. Just as there are good and bad surgeons, there are good and bad lay-therapists, and good and bad medically trained ones.

◊ Checklist

To ensure that you get a good therapist follow the tips below:

☐ Ask your doctor to recommend someone. G.P.s are often very interested in alternative therapies, and many of them have tried one or several themselves. In any case, it is a good idea to let your G.P. know if you are having some form of alternative treatment.

☐ Ask friends, neighbors, or colleagues to recommend someone they have found to be helpful.

☐ Select a practitioner who is registered with one of the alternative professional organizations—at the moment this is your only safeguard that the practitioner you are going to has attained a certain professional standard.

☐ If you have a particular complaint, such as endometriosis, for example, contact one of the self-help organizations to see which therapies might be helpful.

☐ Join or form a self-help group (if there is a branch of the American Holistic Medical Association in your area this would be a good one) to find out what approaches are useful for what problem.

☐ Contact the practitioner you have chosen to see if he or she has treated your condition before. See if you can speak to people who have been treated to find out how satisfied they were.

☐ Don't expect miracles. Sometimes the best any practitioner can do is to help you live with your condition.

☐ Don't expect an instant cure. Most alternative therapies are gentle and take a while to work. The longer you've had a complaint the longer it will take to obtain relief.

☐ Find out beforehand how much you can expect to pay.

☐ Avoid practitioners who claim to have the only answer. A combination of approaches, orthodox and alternative, often works best.

☐ Avoid any practitioner who blames you entirely for your illness.

☐ Look for someone you like and get along with, and who will listen to you and involve you in your treatment.

☐ Do remember that orthodox medicine may be what is appropriate in your particular case. Alternative therapies seem to work best for chronic ailments, self-limiting illnesses, and illnesses with a strong psychological component.

How Can Alternative Therapies Help?

1. They can help you stay well by drawing attention to the effects of your life on your health (e.g., diet, exercise, stress).

2. They can help you deal with chronic disease and help alleviate some of the more troublesome problems.

3. If you become ill they can treat and even cure specific illnesses by helping to put the body's own self-healing mechanisms into action.

4. By putting the emphasis on health rather than disease they can help you increase your sense of positive control over your life.

For further information, contact:

The American Holistic Medical Association/Foundation
2727 Fairview Avenue East
Seattle, WA 98102
(206) 322-6842

Education and research in many areas of alternative medicine, including acupuncture, nutrition, behavioral medicine, and clinical ecology. Offers referrrals to holistic MD's nationwide.

The International Association of Holistic-Health Practitioners
3419 Thom Boulevard
Las Vegas, NV 89106
(702) 873-4542

Worldwide referral service for holistic health centers and practitioners. Public education and research.

Nutritional Therapies

In the last few years the orthodox medical world has begun to sit up and take notice of the role diet has to play in health. Ideas that just a decade ago would have been dismissed as cranky or absurd have become part of the mainstream. It's surely a measure of how far we have come that an article on paleolithic diet (stone age) based on whole food principles should appear in the most prestigious medical journal, *The New England Journal of Medicine.*

♫ Naturopathy

Traditional naturopathy sees acute illness as the body's attempt to rid itself of toxins and return to homeostatis. Much chronic illness is thought to originate from violation of the laws of healthy diet and life-style, and the subsequent mismanagement and suppression of the acute disease process.

The basic tenet of naturopathy is that a healthy diet and life-style can help prevent much illness from occurring in the first place, and that if illness does occur such principles will allow the body's own restorative processes to get to work. According to the naturopath the basic causes of disease can be divided into four groups:

1. *Chemical.* Nutritional deficiency or excess can cause imbalances in the body, leading to poor functioning of lungs, kidneys, and bowels, or poor circulation of body fluids.

2. *Mechanical.* Tight muscles, strained ligaments, and stiff joints or poor posture perhaps because of work, or because the spine is out of balance, lead to problems of functioning for the nervous system and musculo-skeletal system.

3. *Psychological.* Stress leads to problems which can affect the whole body.

4. *Heredity.* While nobody can control her heredity, it is extremely important in determining your basic strengths and weaknesses. It pays to choose healthy parents! You can, however, by the way you live, either make the best of a poor heredity or make the worst of a good one.

The naturopath stimulates the body to heal itself by helping it to get rid of poisons that may have built up. He or she also seeks to help you understand why you became ill in the first place, so that you can take more responsibility for your own health and avoid, where possible, the things that have caused you to become ill. Your first visit to a naturopath will probably be much along the lines of a visit to an orthodox doctor, except that it will be much longer. Blood tests, X rays, and more unconventional methods of diagnosis such as radionics, and iridology may be used, depending on the practitioner.

Treatment includes one or more of the following:

⌗ A *fast*, designed to clear out wastes. This should only be carried out under supervision.

⌗ A *diet* consisting largely of raw foods, unrefined carbohydrates, and a small amount of protein. This may be a type of vegetarian diet, depending on your therapist.

⌗ *Hydrotherapy*—literally water-treatment. This can include applications of hot and cold water, either externally or internally in the form of baths, packs, compresses, sprays, and douches, or sitz baths in which the lower half of the body is immersed in hot or cold water, while the feet are put in water of a contrasting temperature.

⌗ *Structural adjustments* by means of manipulation or massage, remedial exercises, or body realignment techniques such as the Alexander technique.

⌗ *Natural hygiene*, i.e., taking care of yourself by physical exercise, relaxation techniques, and a positive approach to life.

While these treatments formed the core of the traditional naturopathic approach, most naturopaths these days also work extensively with vitamin therapy and herbology. Many include homeopathics and the techniques of the clinical ecologist in their armamentarium, and some do acupuncture or hypnotherapy. Many naturopaths specialize in a certain technique or area, so don't expect them all to use the same treatment or approach to your problem.

Naturopathy can be used for virtually any condition, either as a mainstay or as an adjunct to other forms of treatment. It corresponds in many ways to the general principles for taking care of yourself outlined in the first part of this book.

For further information:

> The American Association of Naturopathic Physicians
> P.O. Box 33046
> Portland, OR 97233
>
> John Bastyr College of Naturopathic Medicine
> 144 N.E. 54th
> Seattle, WA 98105
> (206) 523-9585
>
> National College of Naturopathic Medicine
> 11231 S.E. Market
> Portland, OR 97216
> (503) 255-4860

Naturopathic Medicine: Treating the Whole Person, Roger Newman Turner (Thorsons).

♫ Megavitamin therapy/optimum nutrition

As we've seen throughout the book, many alternative practitioners believe that a large number of illnesses and disorders are a result of excesses or deficiencies of certain important vitamins and minerals. It's important to get the right amount for you personally, since people's needs vary. Megavitamin therapy is said to be especially useful for all those vague aches and pains, chronic tiredness, and lack of energy that afflict so many of us today, as well as menstrual problems, cancer, and even mental disorders. This form of treatment is generally used in conjunction with other therapies by naturopaths, clinical ecologists, and holistic medical physicians.

For further information:

The Whole Health Guide to Elemental Health, Patrick Holford (Thorsons).

The Vitamin Bible, Earl Mindell (Arlington).

Nutrition Almanac, John D. Kirschman (McGraw-Hill).

⚶ Clinical ecology

This is one of the newer approaches, partaking of both orthodox and alternative ideas. Clinical ecologists maintain that many of us are sensitive to certain foods or substances in our environment. Because of the increased use of chemicals in food, and in the environment, such sensitivities are thought to be on the increase. These can be responsible for a wide range of conditions, including the everyday aches and pains, excessive fatigue, irritability, and so on, that all too many of us take for granted. More serious problems such as yeast infections, headaches, migraine headaches, bladder problems, and certain psychological disorders may be triggered by sensitivities to foods, chemicals, or environmental allergens.

A major problem, according to clinical ecologists, is "masked or hidden sensitivity." In other words most of us don't have any obvious reaction to the offending substances. It's only after a fast that a rapid and often dramatic reaction can be provoked. What's more, claim such practitioners, most of us are hooked on the very foods that are making us ill.

Diagnosis

This may involve objective testing such as scratch testing or IgG or IgE RAST testing, or having the patient ingest or inhale small amounts of the suspected allergen and watching the result. Allergy elimination diets, where the person avoids certain foods for a short period and then reintroduces them one at a time, are also used.

Treatment

This may consist of reducing your exposure to offending substances, cutting out foods you are allergic to from your diet, rotating your diet so that you don't eat the remaining foods repetitively and possibly cause more allergies, and desensitization. Many clinical ecologists also try to help you improve your life-style so that you can reduce stress and optimize your nutrition to help you withstand the stress you can't avoid. They also look at the possibility of chronic infections such as candida as possible contributors to your state of increased sensitivity.

For further information:

> The American Academy of Environmental Medicine
> P.O. Box 16106
> Denver, CO 80216
> (303) 622-9755

Clinical Ecology, George Lewith and Julian Kenyon (Thorsons).

Food Allergy: A Primer for People, S. Allen Bock (AJ Publishing Co.).

Herbalism

Herbs have been used for medicine throughout the ages and in every culture. The Chinese, Indians, and Native Americans all have well-developed forms of herbal medicine, and indeed the orthodox pharmocopeia includes many drugs which have their origins in herbs. Herbalism also seems to have a particular attraction for women, perhaps because, as Barbara Ehrenreich and Deirdre English point out in *Witches, Midwives and Nurses: A History of Women Healers* (Writers and Readers):

"Women have always been healers... They were pharmacists, cultivating healing herbs and exchanging the secrets of their uses. They were midwives travelling from home to home and village to village. For centuries, women were doctors without degrees, barred from books and lectures, learning from each other, and passing on experience from neighbor to neighbor and mother to daughter."

Because herbs are there for the picking in every field and hedge it is tempting to treat yourself. And it's true that herbal remedies can provide simple self-help treatments for many minor ailments, *if you know what you are doing.* If you are interested in pursuing this we'd advise that you read *Medicinal Botany I: From the Shephard's Purse,* written and published by Max Barlow, or

Health from God's Garden by Maria Treben, published by Thorsons. But you would be unwise to try and treat yourself for anything that doesn't clear up quickly that you would normally take to the doctor.

An herbalist needs to know not just the symptoms and treatment of illnesses, but which paticular herb to use, what part (leaves, berries, root, bark), how to prepare and apply it, even what time of day to harvest it. Judgment is also needed as to how much to give. Even conventional medicines affect two different people differently, and this is even more marked with herbs. It's far too important a decision to be left to guesswork. Remember, too, that if you're already taking a prescribed or over-the-counter remedy, the herbal treatment could well affect its action in some way.

Herbal treatments work on you and not just on your symptoms, so two entirely different remedies might be given to treat the same disorder. That's why although we've included a few self-help tips later on in the book, you would be advised to consult a proper herbalist or naturopath.

Herbal treatments are extremely effective, because unlike orthodox drugs which take one active ingredient and synthesize it, the whole plant is used. So, while some conventional diuretics, for instance, rob your body of potassium, creating other imbalances in your system, dandelion, a frequently used herbal diuretic, contains large amounts of potassium to counterbalance this effect. Herbal treatments are gentle, unlike modern drugs which are aggressive in their action. They provide trace elements and vitamins as well as active ingredients for a particular condition, which help you to return to full health. So whereas you may feel run-down and washed-out after a conventional course of treatment, after an herbal treatment you may feel full of energy.

⚂ What disorders can herbalism treat?

Many women's ailments can be successfully treated by herbal methods. Painful menstruation and heavy and irregular periods can all be helped. At first, a course of the appropriate medicine can be used with extra medication during your period. Where a hormone imbalance is suspected of being the cause, herbs can be used to correct it, and in this case treatment will probably go on for about six months. There are usually no side effects and you will most likely notice some improvement after one or two cycles. Premenstrual syndrome is very well treated by herbs, and usually needs about three to six months of treatment. PMS symptoms such as migraines may take a little longer to respond, but results are often good. Some vaginal infections can be successfully treated by using a combination of herbal douches, suppositories, and dietary changes. Some cases of infertility due to hormone imbalance can respond to herbal treatment. Menopause discomforts such as hot flashes and vaginal dryness can be helped with herbs that improve hormone balance. Mastitis, cystitis, and irritable bladder can all be treated. For bladder problems, soothing and antiseptic herbs are used, often in the form of herb teas. Herbs can also treat many of the minor ailments of pregnancy safely, and raspberry leaf tea is well known for its effect on toning up the uterus in preparation for labor. Postnatal depression can also be helped.

For further information, contact:

American Herb Association
P.O. Box 353
Rescue, CA 95672
(916) 626-5046

Information and research on herbal products. Publishes directories of mail-order herb sources.

✄ To make an herbal compress

Use a clean muslin or cotton cloth and soak in a hot infusion or decoction. Place it on the affected area and change it when it cools down.

A poultice is similar to a compress except that you use the plant itself. Place either fresh or dried herbs between some muslin and apply to the affected parts. Dried herbs should first be made into a paste, using hot water.

✄ Using an herbal douche

Buy a douche bag at your local drugstore. Use an infusion or decoction which has been allowed to cool. To get the best results, take the douche lying down in the bathtub so that the solution doesn't run out immediately. Let a small amount of liquid enter your vagina and then hold it in by holding the labia together with your hand for a few seconds. Release and repeat until you have used the entire contents of the bag.

NOTE: **NEVER douche if you are pregnant.**

Aromatherapy

Aromatherapy is the use of essential oils derived from aromatic plants and trees for healing. There are about sixty main oils in common use. The oils are either taken by mouth, added to your bathwater, used for massage, inhaled, or given as compresses, douches, or enemas. They are especially useful for stress-related illnesses and infections, either as an adjunct to conventional or alternative therapies or used alone. Be extremely careful when using essential oils. Many are very irritating if not greatly diluted, and sensitivity varies from person to person. Also, they should not be used by people being treated with homeopathics, as they will tend to neutralize the remedy. It's best not to treat yourself, but to consult a qualified practitioner.

For further information:

Aroma Vera Inc.
P.O. Box 3609
Culver City, CA 90231
(213) 973-4253

Oils from organically grown plants.

Essentials
R.D. #2 Box 160A
Ghent, NY 12075
(518) 672-4519

Products based on aromatherapy; therapeutic blends.

Ledet Aromatic Oils
P.O. Box 2354
Fair Oaks, CA 95628
(916) 965-7546

Essential and massage oils; astrological blends.

The Power of Holistic Aromatherapy, Christine Stead (Javeline). Useful self-help guide for a number of minor ailments.

The Art of Aromatherapy Robert Tisserand (Destiny Books).

Bach Flower Remedies

Dr. Edward Bach believed that the cause of any physical illness was a negative emotional state. He claimed that by working on these emotional states by means of the essential energy in certain flowers, many physical ailments could be overcome. The method of preparation involved "placing the flower heads on the surface of water in a plain glass bowl in full sunlight for three hours" then bottling it. The thirty-eight remedies, which you can get from a health food store, are dropped into water and drunk. It all sounds fantastic, but one practitioner who uses Bach Flower Remedies in conjunction with counseling, reflexology, and visualization techniques claims they can be a useful backup to these other methods. Because they are completely harmless they can be safely used for children and babies. A useful remedy is the Rescue remedy, a combination of five Bach Flower Remedies used for "panic, shock; sorrow, terror, sudden bad news, and accidents."

For further information, contact:

The Dr. Bach Healing Society
644 Merrick Rd.
Lynbrook, NY 11563
(516) 593-2206

Homeopathy

Homeopathy works on the principle that "similar cures similar." Remedies made from substances such as herbs, salts, minerals, and even diseased tissue or discharges (nosodes) are used in microscopic dilutions. The idea is that giving minute doses of a medicine that would, in a healthy person, produce the symptoms of the illness being treated stimulates the body's own curative processes. And if that sounds crazy think of X rays, which are known to both cause and cure cancer, or vaccines, which raise resistance to that particular illness.

There are various homeopathic first-aid and self-help remedies, and any of the suppliers listed will be happy to provide lists of the most common ones. However, like herbalism, it would be unwise to try and treat yourself for any but the most simple ailments. There are several books on the market at the moment, which give listed remedies for various women's ailments. Some are useful, but others are too confusing and worse than useless to the uninitiated.

Homeopathic remedies are prescribed for the individual. A homeopath will spend a great deal of time building up a detailed total picture of you as a person and your particular symptoms.

What happens when you visit a homeopath?

Expect to spend about an hour and a half on your first consultation. The homeopath will take a careful history of your symptoms, but will also ask you what you might consider to be some pretty strange questions, such as "Do you prefer to be by the seaside or up in the mountains? "What sort of weather do you prefer?" He or she will also want to know about your family medical history and will ask you about events in your emotional life, such as whether you have suffered a bereavement and how it affected you. Your homeopath will want details too about outside factors that affect your symptoms—for instance, is your illness better when it is warm or cold? All these seemingly unrelated factors are taken into account when prescribing a remedy.

How long will it be before I get better?

Sometimes a single remedy will clear up not just the signs and symptoms of the illness you have gone to the homeopath with, but other ailments or conditions you might not have mentioned. A homeopath told us the story of a woman who had tennis elbow; two weeks afterwards she called up to say that a splinter of glass that had been in her skin for two years had worked its way out too. Sometimes there may be temporary worsening of your condition before you experience any improvement. This is considered to be a sign that the remedy is working. In the case of a long-standing illness it may be necessary to continue giving the same treatment for some time, or to change the remedy as symptoms change. In cases where irreversible bodily changes have already taken place, other types of treatment, or even surgery, may be advised, followed up by homeopathy.

What disorders can homeopaths treat?

Homeopathy can successfully treat most women's ailments, even cysts and fibroids, though these may need surgery. Some cases of cystitis and vaginal discharge may need antibiotics or conventional treatment. But homeopathy may be especially successful for bladder infections that have proved resistant to conventional treatments. Menstrual problems, headaches, and problems associated with menopause can also be treated, as can stress-associated states such as anxiety and depression.

Treatment is in the form of slightly sweet, pleasant tasting pills, powders, or drops. There are homeopathic ointments and creams for external use.

⚘ How does homeopathy work?

⚘ For self help for everyday ailments take the sixth potency.

⚘ For acute conditions take every two hours for two days, then three times daily betwen meals for three days.

⚘ For chronic conditions take three times a day between meals until you feel relief. When you feel some improvement, decrease the number of doses, and stop altogether once you have felt significant

improvement.

⚘ Store medicines away from direct light and strong smelling substances such as toothpaste, perfume, and disinfectants.

⚘ Take medicines in a "clean" mouth. Allow half an hour after eating or cleaning your teeth or smoking a cigarette.

⚘ Don't handle tablets, and if any are spilled don't reuse them.

Sceptics always ask how such infinitesimal doses can work. The short answer is: we don't know. Clinical trials of homeopathic treatment are exceptionally difficult to design, since the same illness will need different remedies depending on the person. However, homeopathy does seem to work, even for children and animals, where the "placebo effect" is hardly likely to account for improvements.

The answer may lie in electromagnetic fields—but so far this hasn't been proved.

⚘ Homeopathy and women

It has to be said that because homeopathy depends so much on subjective views of individuals, there can be a danger of stereotyping. Homeopaths sometimes speak of their patients in terms of their remedies. You'll hear them saying, "She's a typical pulsatilla," for instance. And because many of the materia medica (the books containing symptoms and remedies used by homeopaths for prescribing) were formulated as much as a hundred years ago, the attitudes toward women can be sexist to say the least. It's especially important, therefore, when choosing a homeopathic practitioner to find one you like, who shares your views.

For further information, contact:

> The International Foundation for Homeopathy
> 2366 East Lake E.
> Seattle, WA 98102
> (206) 324-8230

> The National Center for Homeopathy
> 1500 Massachusetts Ave. N.W.
> Suite 41
> Wasington, DC 20005
> (202) 223-6182

Biochemic Tissue Salts

German homeopathic physician Dr. W. H. Schuessler put forward the view that disease was linked to an imbalance of essential minerals. He believed that the body contains twelve essential minerals salts; if these become imbalanced disease results. A dose of the appropriate remedy restores health. The twelve tissue salts are available from most health food stores and can be used for self help. Instructions are usually given on the container, and they are quite easy to use. The twelve salts are as follows:

1. Calcium Fluoride (Calc. Fluor.)
2. Calcium Phosphate (Calc. Phos.)
3. Calcium Sulphate (Calc. Sulph.)
4. Phosphate of Iron (Ferr. Phos.)
5. Potassium Chloride (Kali. Mur.)
6. Potassium Phosphate (Kali. Sulph.)
7. Potassium Sulphate (Kali. Sulph.)
8. Magnesium Phosphate (Mag. Phos.)
9. Sodium Chloride (Nat. Mur.)
10. Sodium Phosphate (Nat. Phos.)
11. Sodium Sulphate (Nat. Sulph.)
12. Silicic Oxide (Silica)

The tissue salts are all given in a minute dose just as in homeopathy. In fact, all of the tissue salts are included in the homeopathic "materia medica," and selection of the remedy is similar though simpler.

For further information: Biochemic Handbook, Colin B. Lessell (Thorsons).

Hands-on Therapies

♫ Osteopathy

Invented by Dr. Andrew Taylor Still in 1874, traditional osteopathy involves correcting structural defects to stimulate healing. The idea is that structural problems such as misalignment of the bones in the spine, muscle spasm, and so on affect nerve and blood flow to other areas of the body, which, if prolonged, can result in disease. Treatment consists of setting right these defects by means of leverage thrusts, stretching, massage, and a variety of other neuromuscular techniques designed to relax the muscles and ligaments and allow the bones to resume their proper position.

Osteopathy is widely accepted by orthodox medicine as a treatment for back pain and other discomfort. Most insurance companies cover osteopathic care. In fact, over the years osteopaths have become so integrated into orthodox medicine that many are indistinguishable from M.D.'s in their practice. Not all osteopaths, by any means, practice traditional osteopathic manipulation. So if this is what you are expecting, ask before you make an appointment.

Visiting an osteopath

A traditional osteopath will look for clues to the underlying cause of your complaint, take special note of your posture and the way you move, and want details about your life and work in order to see if these are causing any particular stresses and strains. The detailed medical history is followed by a physical examination of your spine. Osteopaths are extremely skilled at detecting minute imbalances in spinal structure. If necessary, X rays and urine or blood tests will also be used to aid diagnosis.

Apart from specific osteopathic treatment, the osteopath will give you advice on exercise and how to use your body to maintain health.

For further information:

To find an osteopath near you, contact your state Osteopathic Medical Association.

♫ Chiropractic

Like ostopathy, chiropractic involves manipulating and adjusting for correction, but treats only the spine. The basis of this school of thought is that the spine protects the spinal cord. If the spine is not in proper alignment it interferes with the nerve supply so that the body cannot function properly. The result is disease.

Chiropractic is useful for a whole range of complaints. Like osteopathy, the most common complaints to be treated are back pain, neck problems, and headaches. A recent study by one of the professional chiropractors' associations showed that patients had also been helped with menstrual problems, insomnia, constipation, and bladder problems. The same survey reported that 80 percent of patients got some help from the treatment.

What happens when you visit a chiropractor?

This is very similar to an osteopathic consultation. The chiropractor will take a full case history and may use X rays to aid diagnosis. A physical examination to detect specifid misalignments is next. Treatment consists of thrusting directly on certain bones, a process called adjustment, with a view to encouraging them to return to their correct positions.

What is the difference between chiropractic and osteopathy?

In traditional chiropractic, only the spine is adjusted by means of specific thrusts to the vertebrae. The purpose is to relieve pinched nerves in the intervertebral foramina, which chiropractors believe is responsible for a large number of conditions. The traditional osteopath may use more leverage and massage to help correct structural defects, and treatment is not limited to the spine. While the osteopath treats structural imbalances by means of levering and twisting the body, the chiropractor treats the bones separately by means of specific thrusts.

For further information, contact:

> The International Chiropractors Association
> 1901 L St. NW, Suite 800
> Washington, DC 20036
> (202) 659-6476

✎ Touch for Health—applied kinesiology

There are many programs that use manual muscle testing to determine muscular weakness and imbalances in the energy systems of the body. Applied kinesiology, which started this concept of health care, was originated by George Goodheart,

D.C., in the early 1960s. Today chiropractors, some clinical ecologists, and other health professionals use it as one of their diagnostic tools.

Touch for Health is the layperson's version of applied kinesiology. It was formulated by John Thie, D.C., in the book *Touch for Health* as a way of helping people take charge of their own health by promoting health care within families and among friends. The technique links the traditional Oriental ideas of energy flow found in acupuncture and acupressure with Western-style muscle testing. The idea is to bring about balance within the body by removing toxins, relieving energy blockages, reducing tension, and enhancing the body's natural healing ability.

Certified Touch for Health instructors are available to teach classes so that you can learn to use the system for yourself. There are also licensed health-care professionals who use the Touch for Health system in their therapy.

For information about chiropractors in your area who use applied kinesiology contact:

ICAK (International College of Applied Kinesiology)
11209 Johnson Drive
P.O. Box 25276
Shawnee Mission, KA 66225
(913) 268-8771

For names of Touch for Health instructors or practitioners in your area contact:

Touch for Health Foundation
1174 North Lake Ave.
Pasadena, CA 91104
(818) 794-1181

Further reading:
Touch for Health, John F. Thie, D.C. (DeVorss & Co.).

The Body Says Yes, Priscilla Kapel (ACS Publications, Inc.).

Acupuncture

Although acupuncture has been practiced in the Orient for over 3,000 years, until recently it has been poorly understood and therefore viewed with skepticism in the West. Today, of all the alternative therapies, acupuncture is the one that seems to be attracting the most serious medical interest. There are

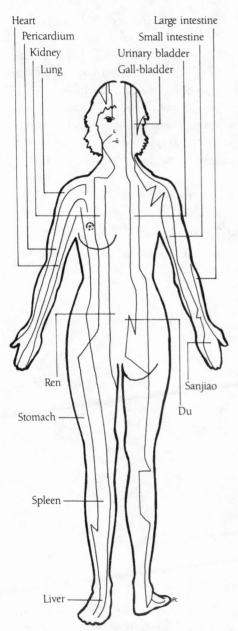

Heart
Pericardium
Kidney
Lung

Large intestine
Small intestine
Urinary bladder
Gall-bladder

Ren
Stomach
Spleen
Liver

Sanjiao
Du

The major acupuncture meridians.

two types of acupuncture being carried out in this country: the traditional Chinese variety, and the modern "scientific" type which relies on scientific explanations of its mode of action.

Chinese medicine, in which acupuncture has its origins, is based on the concept that health is the balance between two opposing forces: Yin (which corresponds to passivity or water) and Yang (which corresponds to activity and is represented by fire). Our body's energy is in a state of constant flux between Yin and Yang—one day we feel fit, the next a bit under the weather. Such change is normal. Illness comes about when these rhythmic changes move too far in one direction or another. Acupuncture attempts to right the balance between Yin and Yang by stimulating acupuncture "points" with fine needles. These points lie along invisible lines, meridians or channels which are said to conduct vital energy or "chi" through the body. The concepts inherent to acupuncture may seem foreign to Westerners, and the idea of chi is hard to explain. Basically it's a bit more than "energy" but a bit less than matter. Blood, food, and gases can be seen as material forms of chi.

Where women's health is concerned, acupuncture can be especially important. In Chinese medicine, for instance, there's a condition known as "empty blood" which can lead to menstrual problems and depression. Treatment is given by means of stimulating points that influence the blood, in order to increase production and aid flow.

Unexpressed emotions or emotional stress are recognized to affect physical problems. A classic acupuncture text, *The Nei Ching*, says that great grief, anxiety, or overthinking may cause a tumor (cancer). Recent scientific thinking about immune mechanisms and their relation to stress is moving conventional medicine nearer to this approach.

However, the properties that have really led to acupuncture being taken into the fold have to do with its pain-relieving effects. It was found in the 1970s that stimulation of the acupuncture points results in the release of endorphins, the body's own pain-relieving substances. Other theories have surmised that acupuncture works by stimulating large nerve fibers, which blocks the pain impulses carried by small nerve fibers (gate control theory). Acupuncture also seems to have a striking effect on the autonomic nervous system. And some recent research points to its anti-inflammatory effect, which could account for its success in treating conditions such as arthritis.

Not all acupuncturists use the traditional system of point selection. Instead, they treat tender points on the skin arising from musculo-skeletal problems. Surprisingly, these points seem remarkably similar to the traditional acupuncture channels.

Diagnosis and treatment

The acupuncturist will spend time detailing your life history, taking note of such factors as your constitution, your emotions, and so on. You'll then be examined to see where any imbalances may lie. On the basis of this he or she will select the appropriate points. Treatment consists of placing needles in these points; the needles remain there from a few seconds to an hour. Sometimes a low-level electric current is applied to the needles, which is thought to encourage endorphin release. It doesn't hurt, though you will probably experience a dull, heavy, or numb feeling or a tingling sensation up and down the meridian.

Symptoms usually disappear gradually, although some people get instant improvement. Your condition may get worse temporarily, but there is no need to worry about this—it's a sign that your body is responding to treatment.

Acupuncture has been found to be effective for 60 percent of chronic pain sufferers, which makes it especially useful for conditions such as endometriosis, headaches, and menstrual pains. It can also be used for childbirth and stress-related disorders such as depression.

There are two main types of acupuncturists—medical doctors, osteopaths, and physical therapists who have taken a course in acupuncture, and traditionally trained and licensed acupuncturists. Your doctor may be able to recommend a trained acupuncturist if he or she is not trained in it.

Ear acupuncture (auricular acupuncture)

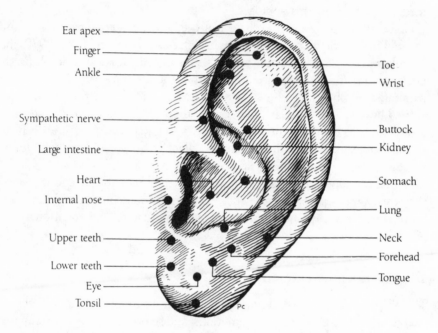

Ear apex
Finger
Ankle
Toe
Wrist
Sympathetic nerve
Large intestine
Buttock
Kidney
Heart
Internal nose
Stomach
Lung
Upper teeth
Lower teeth
Neck
Forehead
Tongue
Eye
Tonsil

Ear acupuncture points.

Parts of the ear are said to correspond to different organs in the body. For instance, if you have a pain in your hand you will experience a pain when the part of your ear corresponding to the hand is pressed. In 70 percent of cases reported in one study, pain could be identified in this way.

For further information, contact:

The Traditional Acupuncture Foundation
American City Building
Suite 100
Columbia, MD 21044
(301) 997-4888

Shiatsu and Acupressure

Shiatsu is the Japanese word meaning finger pressure. It's the Japanese form of acupressure, which follows the same principles as acupuncture, but instead of needles, a form of massage using thumbs, hands, elbows, and even the knees and feet is used to rebalance the body's energy.

Treatments may last anywhere from one-half to one and one-half hours and generally take place once a week, but may be needed more or less frequently depending on the condition. You may be treated sitting, kneeling, or lying down.

Shiatsu is one of the fastest growing alternative therapies. It's also a simple, easy to learn self-help technique that can be used in the home for minor ailments such as headaches and period pains, or as a preventive treatment.

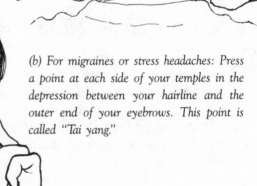

Shiatsu self-help techniques.

(a) For the relief of stress or tension headaches: Massage the points of the back of the neck just below the base of the skull in the depression about one inch on either side of the spine. This point is called "Feng chi."

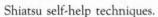

(b) For migraines or stress headaches: Press a point at each side of your temples in the depression between your hairline and the outer end of your eyebrows. This point is called "Tai yang."

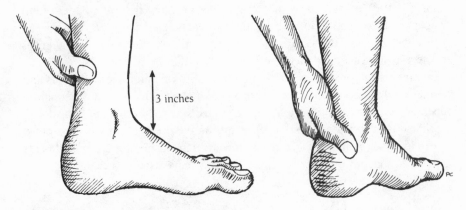

(c) For relief of menstrual pains: Massage the point located four fingers above the inside ankle bone, just behind the shin bone. This point is usally very tender, and is called "San yin jiao."

For further information, contact:

The American Shiatsu Association
Box 718
Jamaica Plain, MA 02130
(617) 522-0251

Reflexology (Zone Therapy/Foot Massage)

Reflexology involves massage of specific points on the hands and feet. Some schools of training emphasize a deep pressure; others teach a lighter touch. It can be done with the fingers or with the aid of tools such as golf balls, pencil erasers, carved wooden probes, or special vibrators. The system is based on the belief that the various organs and tissues of the body are linked reflexively to areas on the feet and hands, and that by stimulation of the nerve endings in these areas you can promote healing in the associated body parts. The practitioner will discover problem areas by feeling small, tender nodules under the skin on the bottom of the foot or the palm of the hand. For instance, if you have a bladder problem, you may feel tenderness in the arch of your foot (the bladder reflex area), or you may experience sensations in your bladder when the therapist massages the part of the arch near your heel.

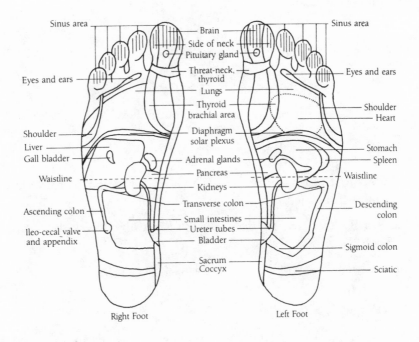

Sinus area — Brain — Sinus area
Side of neck
Pituitary gland
Eyes and ears — Threat-neck, thyroid — Eyes and ears
Lungs
Thyroid brachial area — Shoulder
Heart
Shoulder — Diaphragm solar plexus
Liver — Stomach
Gall bladder — Adrenal glands — Spleen
Waistline — Pancreas — Waistline
Kidneys
Transverse colon — Descending colon
Ascending colon — Small intestines
Ileo-cecal valve and appendix — Ureter tubes
Bladder — Sigmoid colon
Sacrum Coccyx — Sciatic

Right Foot   Left Foot

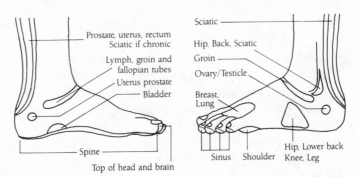

Prostate, uterus, rectum
Sciatic if chronic
Lymph, groin and fallopian tubes
Uterus prostate
Bladder

Sciatic
Hip, Back, Sciatic
Groin
Ovary/Testicle
Breast, Lung

Spine
Top of head and brain

Sinus   Shoulder   Hip, Lower back
Knee, Leg

Reflex zones of the feet.

Reflexology can be extremely relaxing and is said to benefit most stress-related disorders. It can help menstrual problems and those related to menopause, as well as headaches and high blood pressure. It is a useful adjunct to other types of therapy or can be used alone. A reflexology practitioner may do only reflexology or may combine it with other therapies such as massage.

For further information:

> Kevin and Barbara Kunz
> Reflexology Research Project
> P.O. Box 35820, Stn. D
> Albuquerque, NM 87176
>
> International Institute of Reflexology
> P.O. Box 12642
> St. Petersburg, FL 3373-2642

Hand and Foot Reflexology, A Self-Help Guide, Kevin and Barbara Kunz (Prentice-Hall, Inc.).

The Foot Book, Healing the Body Through Reflexology, Devaki Berkson (Harper & Row Publishers, Inc.).

Reflexology: A Patient's Guide, Nicola Hall (Thorsons).

Massage

Massage was mentioned by Hippocrates as a healing art, and has been practiced in the Far East for thousands of years. It's a simple, pleasurable way to ease aches and pains, aid relaxation, and combat stress. Athletes use it to improve their performance or to shorten the healing time of injuries. Anyone can give a friend a simple back rub, but specialized training is necessary for someone who wants to do therapeutic massage professionally.

When you go for a massage, you can expect the therapist to use a combination of stroking (effleurage), rubbing, kneading, percussion, and point pressure. He or she may use specially scented oils or lotions. You will be kept warm and draped at all times. If you have an injury, the therapist may also use hot or cold packs before or after treatment.

Of course, there is no need to be ill or injured to enjoy a massage, but it can be useful if you are suffering from some illnesses or injuries. In England certain hospitals now include it as part of their therapy for patients who have had a heart attack, and many European sports teams have a massage therapist who travels with them during competitions.

To find a suitable masseuse, start by asking people you know. A personal recommendation is your best guarantee. Next try local gyms and health clubs and even beauty parlors—many of them have a resident massage practitioner. If you have to resort to the Yellow Pages, call first and ask if the massage therapist is a member of the American Massage Therapy Association, the national professional organization. Its members must meet high educational, moral, and professional standards.

The Massage Book, by George Downing (Penguin), is full of useful hints if you want to learn to massage. Here are some of them:

___ Apply enough pressure when you massage.

___ Keep your hands relaxed.

___ Mold your hands to fit the contours of your partner's body.

___ Maintain steady speed and pressure.

___ Explore the underlying structure of your partner's body.

___ Use your weight rather than muscle power to apply pressure.

___ Keep in continuous contact with your partner's body throughout the massage.

___ Massage with your whole body, not just your hands.

___ Don't strain yourself.

___ Remember your partner is a person and not just a piece of dough!

___ Ask your partner what he or she likes best.

For further information:

American Massage Therapy Association
P.O. Box 1270
Kingsport, TN 37662

Sports Massage, Jack Meagher and Pat Boughton (Dolphin Books, Doubleday and Co., Inc.).

New Massage: Total Body Conditioning for People Who Exercise, Gordon Inkeles (Perigee Books, The Putnam Publishing Group).

Alexander Technique

The Alexander technique, named after its founder, F. Matthias Alexander, is an educational process designed to bring about easy movement and improved coordination. It is a way to free yourself of old habits and to gain conscious control of how you move. Practitioners claim that as you rid yourself of the physical stress that results from misuse of your body, you also find that your general health gets better and that many daily aches and pains disappear.

The technique may be taught privately or in groups. You learn general principles and how to apply them to your specific needs. During a series of lessons, you discover that in any movement the relationship between your head, neck, and whole body is of primary importance to the way in which you move. You increase your awareness of old habits of movement in simple activities like sitting or walking, and in more complex ones such as dancing, playing a musical instrument, working at a computer, or diapering a baby. You learn to stop automatically moving in your habitual ways. Then you experiment with new ways of moving which improve your performance within these same activities. By changing the way you think about how you move, you change your movement.

For further information:

The Use of the Self, F. Matthias Alexander (Centerline Press).

Body Awareness in Action: A Study of the Alexander Technique, Frank Pierce Jones (Schocken Books).

On teachers: The listings below represent a variety of methods of teaching the Alexander technique. You will not get the same list of names from every organization, so if you want to see if you have a choice of teachers in your area, contact all five groups.

American Center for the Alexander Technique
1913 Thayer Ave.
Los Angeles, CA 90025

North American Society of Teachers of the Alexander Technique
810 Broadway, Suite 2
New York, NY 10003

Society of Teachers of the Alexander Technique
10 London House
266 Fulham Rd.
London, SW 10 9EL
United Kingdom

The F.M. Alexander School
610 W. Phil-Ellen St.
Philadelphia, PA 19119

The Performance School
6836 21st N.E.
Seattle, WA 98115

Movement Therapies

♫ Yoga

Yoga doesn't fall easily into the category of a therapy as such. Even so, it benefits every aspect of the body, mind, and spirit, which makes it useful as an adjunct to almost any other type of treatment, and also a particularly beneficial form of exercise. The physical practice of yoga consists of asanas (postures) and breathing exercises (pranayama). But yoga is far more than just a system of exercise. The four paths of yoga are:

1. action
2. devotion
3. knowledge and wisdom
4. physical and mental control

Hatha yoga is the type most commonly practiced in the West. The emphasis in a yoga class will vary according to your teacher, but at least at first the emphasis is on physical and mental control. Once you've learned the techniques you can practice them regularly at home. Yoga is especially useful for combatting and avoiding the effects of stress, which makes it a valuable preventive and treatment for almost any illness.

For further information:

There is no national yoga association in the United States, but every year the July/August edition of *Yoga Journal* magazine lists yoga teachers throughout the country.

Yoga Journal
2054 University Ave.
Berkeley, CA 94704

Further reading: Light on Yoga, B.K.S. Iyengar (Schocken Books).

∬ T'ai Chi Ch'uan

T'ai Chi, as it's more usually known, is a form of movement meditation through a sequence of gentle, flowing actions. In fact if you see T'ai Chi in action it's hard to believe that it is in fact a martial art. Above all, T'ai Chi is slow and gentle. It exercises every part of the body, and leads to an increased sense of well-being and tranquility. Because it is nonaggressive it is especially attractive to women and older people or heart patients for whom more active types of movement would be unsuitable.

While there is no national T'ai Chi Ch'uan organization in the U.S., teachers are available in most large cities and in many smaller communities as well. Contact a local health club, dance studio, or martial arts organization for information on T'ai Chi schools in your area.

∬ Dance/movement therapy

Dance has been part of human celebration and healing for thousands of years. It can be a powerful form of expression and creativity, integrating the physical, emotional, and spiritual aspects of oneself. Dance/movement therapy attempts to combine the function and expression of the body with the mental and emotional state of the person. The therapy is said to be especially helpful in deepening one's sense of the physical self and in promoting growth toward mind/body unity.

There are many different approaches to dance/movement therapy. Some therapists focus more on expression, creativity, and the artistic properties inherent in dance. Others emphasize the more functional aspects of body movement. Which method you choose will depend on your issues and interests.

Dance/movement therapy is claimed to be particularly suited to people who want to "be in their body" and release the muscular and energetic "holding" that can prevent freedom of movement and emotional expression.

For further information contact:

The American Dance Therapy Association
2000 Century Plaza
Columbia, MD 21044

Mind Therapies

∬ Psychotherapy

Psychotherapy includes any treatment that uses talking instead of drug treatment. It may be given by a psychiatrist, a medically trained doctor with extra training in psychology, or a psychologist, who has made a study of the mind and its mechanisms.

There are many different approaches to psychotherapy, and it's clearly impossible in a book such as this to go into them all.

A useful rundown of psychotherapeutic techniques that are commonly used, and can be used as the basis of self-help groups, is to be found in *In Our Own Hands* by Sheila Ernst and Lucy Goodison (Women's Press). Because of the many different approaches to psychotherapy, it's important to find someone you feel happy with and trust.

It's not easy finding a psychotherapist. You could try asking your doctor; most physicians have one or more therapists whom they trust and will refer you to. Friends may also know someone whom they have found helpful.

There is no central referral service for psychotherapy, as the approaches vary widely. Each of the various disciplines has schools and associations who will refer you to practitioners in your area.

∬ Hypnotherapy

Hypnosis is an altered state of mind. A hypnotist I spoke to described being hypnotized as being akin to the sensation you experience in the moment between sleeping and waking. The hypnotherapist enables this state be extended, which makes it a useful way to "unlock" the mind, and therefore it works very well as a form of psychotherapy. You can also be trained to hypnotize yourself (autohypnosis), which can be a useful technique for dealing with stress, pain, and so on.

People are often worried that under hypnotism they will be persuaded to do things they wouldn't normally do in everyday life, a fear which is fueled by the use of hypnotism as a form of popular entertainment. The hypnotist I spoke to assured me that this couldn't happen, and that you would automatically snap out of the hypnotic state if you were asked to do something you didn't agree to. However, it has to be said that research in this area is contradictory, so be careful who you go to.

Hypnotherapy can be useful in helping you give up smoking, come off tranquilizers, cope with the pain of childbirth, and relieve anxiety, depression, headaches, and migraine. A recent report in a medical journal shows it to be effective for some women experiencing repeated miscarriages.

People vary in how suggestible they are, and hypnotherapy doesn't work for everyone. Where it does, it can help you deal with problems that are troubling you faster than ordinary psychotherapy by bypassing the barriers we normally put up to defend ourselves against facing troublesome issues.

In fact, one of the potential problems with hypnotherapy is that too much of what is troubling you can be brought up at once. Hypnotherapists must be careful not to overwhelm their clients by helping them to remember more than they can handle at the time.

Many orthodox doctors have now learned hypnotism, and your G.P. may be willing to refer you to a reputable nonmedical practitioner.

For further information:

American Counsel of Hypnotism Examiners
312 Riverdale Dr.
Glendale, CA 91204
(818) 242-1159

Miracles on Demand: The Radical Short-Term Therapy of Gil Boyne, Charles Tebbets (Westwood Publishers).

♫ Co-counseling—re-evaluation counseling

This is a particularly useful therapy for helping you to deal with problems that are bothering you, problems that perhaps aren't serious enough to warrant professional psychotherapy. Two people take it in turns to counsel each other, trading off the roles of client and counselor.

You have to take a special sixteen week introduction course that teaches you a few simple listening techniques, and gives you practice at remaining relaxed in the face of another person discharging tensions. You will also learn how the processes of emotional discharge and re-evaluation operate. The basic idea is that by throwing off the restraints normally placed on the expression of feeling by your upbringing—through laughter, tears, trembling, anger (catharsis)—you can let go of things from your past that prevent you from living in the present, and help you to better understand yourself and your relationships with others.

Its present focus makes it a very positive type of therapy which is especially suitable for women, since the normal power structure that operates between helper and helped is shared between counselor and client.

Those participating in re-evaluation counseling do not advise each other, and those people who are severely distressed may need professional counseling first before they can effectively use re-evaluation counseling.

For further information contact:

Personal Counselors, Inc.
719 Second Ave. North
Seattle, WA 98109
(206) 284-0311

Personal Counselors puts out a magazine called *Present Time*, which talks about issues in re-evaluation counseling and gives names of people who are co-counselors nationally and internationally.

♫ Autogenic training

This is a well-established, effective relaxation method developed in Germany by C. Schultz and Hans Luthe. It is basically a form of autohypnosis that can help you give up alcohol or smoking; deal with depression, tension, hostility, premenstrual tension, and menopausal problems; and help you come off tranquilizers, sleeping tablets, and other drugs.

For further information:

Handbook of Innovative Psychotherapy, Raymond Corsini (Wiley and Sons).

Relieve Tensions the Autogenic Way, Hannes Lindemann (Peter H. Wyden).

♫ Biofeedback

Biofeedback is not a therapy as such, but can be used to aid relaxation, yoga, and autogenic training. It's a way of monitoring bodily processes such as blood pressure, heart rate, temperature, and muscle tension by means of a biofeedback machine. The machine is usually a little electronic box which gives out a continuous tone or bleep. Two electrodes which measure changes in the body's surface moisture are attached to the palms of your hands. The premise is that when you feel tense or anxious you sweat more—think of the clammy hands you get when you visit the dentist! The machine picks up minute changes in body moisture and the tone emitted rises; when you are calm it falls. In this way you can figure out when you are really relaxed.

Biofeedback has found great favor in the medical community as a stress-relieving technique. It is often suggested as a treatment for elevated blood pressure, when stress appears to be a major component of the problem. You can also use it if you suffer from tension headaches, backaches, or any other complaint where stress is a component. Biofeedback has also been quite successful when used in the treatment of certain neurological disorders and injuries.

For further information, contact:

The Biofeedback Society of America
10200 W. 44th Avenue, Suite 304
Wheat Ridge, CO. 80033
303/422-8436

Many larger cities have at least one biofeedback clinic, often associated with a hospital. Your doctor will probably be able to refer you to a clinic in your area.

Further reading:

Mind as Healer, Mind as Slayer, Kenneth Pelletier (Peter Smith Publishers, Inc.).

Your Body: Biofeedback as Its Best, Beate Jencks (Nelson-Hall, Inc.).

♫ Spiritual healing

The ritual of "laying on of hands" is as old as the human race, and the belief that some people are able to tap into a healing force that can be channeled from the healer to the sick person is not a new one. Spiritual healing doesn't always involve the "laying on of hands"; it can also be done at a distance.

How does it work?

According to Brian Inglis and Ruth West in *The Alternative Health Guide* (Michael Joseph): "The hypothesis is that healers have something in their 'energy field' which is capable of interacting with and replenishing the energy fields of patients. How this happens remains a mystery."

It all sounds too fantastic to be true. Nonetheless, throughout the ages there have been anecdotal reports of people being mysteriously healed after contact with a healer.

Two types of spiritual healing which have recently gained in popularity are Reiki and therapeutic touch. The Reiki sytem as practiced today originated in the 1800s with Dr. Mikao Usui, a Japanese educator. After extensive study of the healing phenomena of some of history's greatest spiritual healers, he evolved a healing system based on ancient Buddhist teachings. Reiki practitioners believe that they attune themselves to the Reiki, or universal life energy, and channel it through themselves to those they are healing. They maintain that Reiki accelerates the healing proces, and gives a feeling of well-being. In the words of Phyllis Lei Furumoto, Reiki Grand Master, this system "opens the mind and spirit to the causes of disease and pain and the necessity for taking responsibility for one's life."

Therapeutic touch, a modern derivative of laying on of hands, has been subjected to trials in America for the treatment of tension headache. The patients who had received TT had an average 70 percent reduction in pain which carried on over the next four hours, which was greater than a group subjected to a placebo.

It seems that, like so many healing processes, spiritual healing and therapeutic touch could work in some way by reducing stress. One researcher in the U.S. demonstrated increased hemoglobin levels in patients following therapeutic touch. Patients who have received healing and therapeutic touch report deep feelings of relaxation. But even where such treatments don't effect a cure, perhaps the feelings of being more relaxed and able to cope count more than anything. An article in the *Nursing Times* has this to say: "After the session, most of the patients said they felt extremely relaxed and more able to cope with day to day problems. Some felt physical pain relief immediately . . . For some the success of the physical healing was not important. They just wanted somebody to listen to their problems.

For further information, contact:

> The Reiki Alliance
> 535 Cordova Rd., Suite 419
> Santa Fe, NM 87501
> (505) 982–5331

Incidentally, you don't have to belong to a religion or have religious faith to benefit from spiritual healing.

⌗ Meditation

The image many of us associate with the word meditation is of someone sitting in a flowing robe contemplating a flower. In fact, there are many different ways of meditating. Concentrating on an object such as a flower, a vase, or a picture is just one. Meditation can incorporate many alternative therapies. Alexander technique and Tai Chi, for instance, can be ways of reaching a meditative state through the use of the body. It's important to find the way of meditating that suits you as an individual.

Meditation has time and again been shown to have physiological effects. Experienced yogis can control their blood pressure, heart rate, and other bodily processes during meditation. And it's recently been shown that meditation has an effect on the immune system. This could explain its usefulness in preventing and treating illness.

With practice, meditation can help you see the world in a new way, and can give you increased energy and enthusiasm. But if you're expecting instant enlightenment, forget it. Holistic doctor Laurence LeShan says in *How to Meditate* (Turnstone): "Insight experiences do occur . . . but they are only the beginning . . . After the insight comes the long hard work of following it up: of changing our perceptions, feelings and behaviour to gradually, painfully, bring them into accord with our understanding."

There are plenty of good books around that can teach you the basics of meditation. Mental meditation, through concentrating on counting your breaths, or a mantra (a phrase that you repeat during the meditation), is perhaps the easiest from of meditation to teach yourself. If your "path of meditation" is through the body, perhaps through dance, yoga, Tai Chi, or the practice of a particular skill such as weaving, pottery, or singing, you will probably need a teacher.

Meditation can also be achieved through your emotions, by "loosening your feelings."

As always, choose a school of meditation or teacher who appeals to you. Beware of charismatic leaders who claim to be the fount of all wisdom, or claim to possess some special secret knowledge.

Tips for meditating

⌗ Work out how much time you have to give to it. Be realistic.

⌗ Set aside a regular period each day—

say fifteen to twenty minutes when you know you won't be disturbed.

⌗ Set aside a place for meditating.

A warm room, where the lighting can be dimmed by drawing the curtains or switching off the light is suitable.

✍ Don't meditate immediately after a meal or after drinking coffee, tea, or alcohol.

✍ Allow yourself a few minutes to come to slowly after meditating.

For further information:

Centering, Sanders Laurie and Melvin Tucker (Destiny).

The Quiet Therapies, David Reynolds (University Press of Hawaii).

Table showing illnesses and therapies

This is only a very rough guide. Some of the illnesses will need orthodox treatment as well as alternative. For more details consult the appropriate sections in the book.

KEY: xxx = excellent results
xx = worth a try
x   = may be useful as an adjunct to other therapies, orthodox or alternative.

Therapies	Acupuncture	Alexander technique	Aromatherapy	Bach flower remedies	Biochemic tissue salts	Biofeedback	Chiropractic	Clinical ecology	Dance therapy	Herbal medicine	Homoeopathy	Hypnotherapy	Massage	Meditation/visualization	Megavitamin therapy	Naturopathy	Osteopathy	Psychotherapy	Reflexology	Shiatsu	Spiritual healing	Yoga
Dysmenorrhea	xxx	x	x		x			x	x	xx	xx	xx	x	xx	x	xx	x	x	x	x		xxx
Depression	xx	xx	xx	xx	x			x	xx	xx	xx	xxx	xx	xxx	xx	xxx	xx	xxx	xx	x	xx	xx
Cystitis				xx	xx			xxx		xxx	xxx			x	xx	xxx	xx		xx			xx
Chlamydia									x	x												
Cervical erosion			x						xx	xx		xx		xx	x	xx			x			
Cancer	x		x						xx	xx	xx		xx	xxx	xxx	xxx		xxx		xxx		
Benign breast disease	xx							xxx		xxx	xx					xxx			x	x		
Bartholin cyst										xx	xx					xxx						
Anxiety	xx	xx	x	xx	x	xxx		xxx	xxx	xxx	xxx	xxx	xxx	xxx	xx	xx	x	xxx	xx	xx		xx
Anemia								xx	xxx	xx												
Amenorrhea	xxx				xx	xx		xx		xxx	xxx	xx		xx	xx	xx	xx		xx		xx	
AIDS	xx									xx				xx	xx	xx		xx			xx	

Therapies	Endometriosis	Fatigue	Fibroids	Headache/migraine	Herpes	Hot flashes	Infertility	Osteoporosis	PID	Postnatal depression	Pre-eclamptic toxemia	Thrush	Trichomonas
Acupuncture	xx	xx	xxx	xxx			xxx			xx			
Alexander technique		xxx		xxx						x			
Aromatherapy		xx		xx	x					x			
Bach flower remedies		x								x			
Biochemic tissue salts													
Biofeedback				xx							xxx		
Chiropractic				xxx									
Clinical ecology	xx	xxx	xxx	xxx			xxx			xx		xx	
Dance therapy		xxx								xx			
Herbal medicine	xxx	x	xxx	xxx	xxx	xxx	xxx	xx	xxx	xx		xxx	xx
Homoeopathy	xxx	x	xx	xxx	xxx	xxx	xxx	xxx	xxx	xx	x	xxx	xx
Hypnotherapy	xx	x		xx			xx			xx	xx		
Massage		x		xxx						xx		x	
Meditation/visualization	xxx	x	xx	xx	xx	x	xx		xx	xx	x	x	x
Megavitamin therapy	xxx	xxx		xx	xx	xxx	xxx	xxx		xxx	x	x	
Naturopathy	xxx	xxx	xxx	xxx	xxx	xxx	xxx	xxx		xxx	xx	xxx	
Osteopathy		xx		xxx			xx			x			x
Psychotherapy				x	x					xxx			
Reflexology	xx	xx	x	xx			x			xx			
Shiatsu	x	xx		xxx									
Spiritual healing		xxx	xx	xxx	xx		xxx			xxx			
Yoga		xxx		xxx						xxx